445-9613

P9-DUS-194

Handbook of Nursing Diagnosis

Second Edition

Lynda Juall Carpenito, R.N., M.S.N.

Nursing Consultant, Mickleton, New Jersey

J. B. Lippincott Company   Philadelphia

London   Mexico City   New York   St. Louis   São Paulo   Sydney

Acquisitions Editor: Diana Intenzo
Sponsoring Editor: Jeanne Wallace
Manuscript Editor: Lee Henderson
Indexer: Barbara Littlewood
Design Director: Tracy Baldwin
Design Coordinator: Don Shenkle
Production Supervisor: Carol A. Florence
Production Coordinator: Kathleen R. Diamond
Compositor: TAPSCO, Inc.
Printer/Binder: R. R. Donnelley & Sons Company

Second Edition

Copyright © 1987, by J. B. Lippincott Company
Copyright © 1985, by J. B. Lippincott Company. All rights
reserved. No part of this book may be used or reproduced in any
manner whatsoever without written permission except for brief
quotations embodied in critical articles and reviews. Printed in
the United States of America. For information write J. B.
Lippincott Company, East Washington Square, Philadelphia,
Pennsylvania 19105.

6 5 4

Library of Congress Cataloging-in-Publication Data

Carpenito, Lynda Juall.
   Handbook of nursing diagnosis.

   Includes index.
   1. Diagnosis—Handbooks, manuals, etc.   2. Nursing—
Handbooks, manuals, etc.   I. Title. [DNLM: 1. Nursing
Process—handbooks. WY 39 C294h]
RT48.C365   1987   616.07′5   86-27439
ISBN 0-397-54654-8

To Olen, my son

for your innocence and wisdom
for our quiet moments and sudden hugs
for your unsolicited distractions
. . . I am grateful

for you are my daily reminder of what is
really important . . .
love, health, and human trust

Introduction

DIAGNOSTIC CATEGORIES

In 1973, the North American Nursing Diagnosis Association (NANDA; formerly, the National Group for the Classification of Nursing Diagnosis) published its first list of nursing diagnoses. Since that time, the interest in nursing diagnosis and its application in clinical settings has grown substantially. In the 1970s, the main issue in nursing centered on the value of establishing a classification system for nursing diagnoses. Now that there is general agreement about the need for a formal taxonomy, the current issue is the implementation of nursing diagnoses. The challenge that nurses face today is one of identifying specific nursing diagnoses for those people assigned to their care and of incorporating these diagnoses into a plan of care.

This handbook does not focus on teaching nurses about the concept of nursing diagnosis. For information describing the concept and specific instructions for clinical use the reader is referred to Carpenito LJ: Nursing Diagnosis: Application to Clinical Practice, 2nd ed. Philadelphia, JB Lippincott, 1987.

This handbook is intended to supplement texts on nursing diagnosis in two ways:

- By providing a quick reference to each diagnostic category in terms of its definition, defining characteristics, and etiological, contributing, and risk factors
- By identifying possible nursing diagnoses and collaborative problems that could be associated with the major medical diagnoses

Section I consists of 72 diagnostic categories, including 65 approved by NANDA and seven additional categories. The additional categories are

Impaired Communication

Health Maintenance

Potential for Infection Transmission

Alterations in Parental Role

Potential Alteration in Respiratory Function

Potential for Self-harm

Maturational Enuresis

Each diagnostic category is described in terms of

- Definition
- Defining characteristics, which are a cluster of signs and symptoms that are separated into major and minor classifications. The *major* category includes those signs and symptoms that must be present to validate use of a diagnosis. The *minor* classification refers to characteristics that appear to be present in many but not all individuals experiencing the diagnosis. Minor characteristics are not less serious than the major ones; they are just not present in all individuals.
- Etiological, contributing, and risk factors, which are examples of pathophysiological, treatment-related, situational, and maturational factors that can cause or influence the health status or contribute to the development of a problem

ACTUAL, POTENTIAL, AND POSSIBLE NURSING DIAGNOSES

A nursing diagnosis can be actual, potential, or possible.

Actual: An actual nursing diagnosis describes a diagnostic category that the nurse has validated because of the presence of major defining characteristics, or signs and symptoms.

Potential: A potential nursing diagnosis describes an altered state that is not present but may occur if certain nursing interventions are not ordered and implemented.

Possible: A possible nursing diagnosis describes a problem that the nurse suspects may be present but that requires additional data collection to confirm or rule out its presence.

DIAGNOSTIC STATEMENTS

The diagnostic statement is a statement that describes the health status of an individual or group and the factors that have contributed to the status.

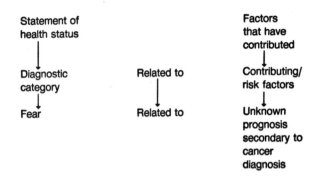

The diagnostic statement or the nursing diagnosis should consist of two or three parts.

Two-part Statements

Potential and possible nursing diagnoses have two parts. The validation for a potential nursing diagnosis is the presence of risk factors. The risk factors are the second part.

Potential nursing diagnosis   Related to   Risk factors

Possible nursing diagnoses are suspected because of the presence of certain factors. The nurse then either rules out or confirms the existence of an actual or a potential diagnosis.

Examples of two-part statements are

Potential Impairment of Skin Integrity related to immobility secondary to fractured hip

Possible Self-care Deficit related to impaired ability to use left hand secondary to IV

Three-part Statements

An actual nursing diagnosis consists of three parts.

Diagnostic label + contributing factors + signs and symptoms

The presence of major signs and symptoms (defining characteristics) validates that an actual diagnosis is present.

It is not possible to have a third part for potential or possible diagnoses because signs and symptoms do not exist.

Examples of three-part statements are

Anxiety related to unpredictable nature of asthmatic episodes as manifested by statements of "I'm afraid I won't be able to breathe."

Urge Incontinence related to diminished bladder capacity secondary to habitual frequent voiding as manifested by inability to hold off urination after desire to void and report of voiding out of habit, not need

The presence of a nursing diagnosis is determined by assessing the individual's health status and his ability to function. To guide the nurse who is gathering this information, a Data-Base Assessment Tool is included in the Appendix at the end of the book. This guide directs the nurse to collect data according to the individual's functional health patterns. Functional health patterns and the corresponding nursing diagnoses are listed in the table that follows this introduction. If significant data are collected in a particular functional pattern, the next step is to check the related diagnostic categories to see if any nursing diagnoses are substantiated by the data that are collected.

Section II of this handbook consists of seven parts: (1) Medical Diagnoses, (2) Surgical Procedures, (3) Obstetric/ Gynecologic Conditions, (4) Neonatal Conditions, (5) Pediatric/Adolescent Disorders, (6) Psychiatric Disorders, and (7) Diagnostic and Therapeutic Procedures. Each of these subjects is represented by a series of major medical diagnoses under which are listed a group of associated nursing diagnoses and collaborative problems. The intent of this section is to help the nurse identify possible nursing diagnoses in each of these areas. It is important to note that each nursing diagnosis must be confirmed or ruled out on the basis of the data collected. The use of a nursing diagnosis without clinical validation based on defining characteristics is hazardous and unsound, and jeopardizes the effectiveness and validity of the nursing care plan. The listing of tentative nursing diagnoses under medical and surgical diagnoses was intended to facilitate the assessment, identification, and validation process, *not to replace it.*

In addition to the potential nursing diagnoses listed under each medical category, there is a list of potential collaborative problems or complications that may occur. Nurses intervene in both types of situations. The first type are called collaborative problems.

Collaborative problems are defined as follows:

Collaborative problems are the physiological complications that have resulted or may result from pathophysiological and treatment-related situations. Nurses monitor to detect their onset or status and collaborate with medical caregivers for definitive treatment.

Examples:

Pathophysiological   *Treatment-related*
Hepatitis   Medications
Stroke   Mechanical ventilation
         → Collaborative problems ←

For collaborative problems, nurses prescribe and implement monitoring interventions that are in the domain of nursing. Monitoring interventions may also be indicated for nursing diagnoses.

The nature of collaborative problems is that they are present or at risk of being present whenever the pathology or treatment is present. For example, all postoperative abdominal surgery clients will be at risk for hemorrhage, hypoxia, and so forth. Expert nursing knowledge will be required to determine who is at risk and to identify these individuals at an early stage to prevent morbidity.

A single format for labeling collaborative problems is needed in order to provide consistency for documentation and computer coding. The following is recommended as a logical way of labeling collaborative problems:

Examples:

Potential complication: (specify)

Potential complication: Arrhythmias

Potential complication: Sepsis

Potential complication: Hypoglycemia

The second type of situation is the nursing diagnosis. Nursing diagnoses represent those areas for which the nurse can legally prescribe the primary interventions. These items are listed according to the formal terminology associated with nursing diagnoses.

Nursing diagnosis is defined as follows:

Nursing diagnosis is a statement that describes the human response (health state or actual/potential altered interaction pattern) of an individual or group that the nurse can legally identify and for which the nurse can order definitive interventions to maintain the health state or to reduce, eliminate, or prevent alterations.

For nursing diagnoses, nurses prescribe interventions that are definitive for prevention and treatment. For collaborative problems, nurses do not prescribe definitive treatment but do prescribe monitoring interventions for early detection. For additional information on nursing diagnoses and collaborative problems, refer to Chapter 2 of Carpenito LJ: Nursing Diagnosis: Application to Clinical Practice, 2nd ed. Philadelphia, JB Lippincott, 1987.

How to Use the Manual

1. Collect data, both subjective and objective, from client, family, other health care professionals, and records. (Refer to Appendix: Adult Data-Base Assessment Guide.)
2. Identify a possible pattern or problem.
3. Refer to the medical diagnostic category and review the possible associated nursing diagnoses and collaborative problems. Select the possibilities.
4. After you have selected what physiological complications or collaborative problems are indicated to be monitored for, label them as Potential complications: (specify)
5. After you have determined which functional patterns are altered or at risk of altered functioning, review the list of nursing diagnostic categories under that pattern and select the appropriate diagnosis. (Refer to Table 1.)
6. If you select an actual diagnosis,
   • Do you have signs and symptoms to support its presence? (Refer to Section I, Nursing Diagnostic Categories, under the selected diagnosis.)

- Write the actual diagnosis in three parts:
      Category related to contributing factors as manifested by signs and symptoms
7. If you select a potential diagnosis
   - Are risk factors present?
   - Write the potential diagnosis in two parts:
      Category related to risk factors
8. If you suspect a problem but have insufficient data, gather the additional data to confirm or rule out the diagnosis. If this additional data collection must be done later or by other nurses, label the diagnosis *possible* on the care plan.*

* Specific focus assessment criteria questions, outcome criteria, and interventions for each nursing diagnosis category can be found in Carpenito LJ: Nursing Diagnosis: Application to Clinical Practice, 2nd ed. Philadelphia, JB Lippincott, 1987.

Table 1. Nursing Diagnostic Categories Grouped Under Functional Health Patterns*

1. Health perception–health management pattern
    Growth and Development, Altered
    † Health Maintenance
    Health Maintenance, Alteration in
    Noncompliance
    Potential for Injury

2. Nutritional–metabolic pattern
    Body Temperature, Potential Altered
    Fluid Volume Deficit
    Fluid Volume Excess
    Infection, Potential for
    † Infection Transmission, Potential for
    Nutrition, Alteration in: Less Than Body Requirements
    Nutrition, Alteration in: More Than Body Requirements
    Swallowing, Impaired
    Thermoregulation, Ineffective
    Tissue Integrity, Impaired
       Oral Mucous Membrane, Alteration in
       Skin Integrity, Impairment of

3. Elimination pattern
    Bowel Elimination, Alteration in: Constipation
    Bowel Elimination, Alteration in: Diarrhea

Bowel Elimination, Alteration in: Incontinence
Urinary Elimination, Alteration in: Patterns of
   Urinary Retention
   Total Incontinence
   Functional Incontinence
   Reflex Incontinence
   Urge Incontinence
   Stress Incontinence
   † Maturational Enuresis

4. Activity–exercise pattern
   Activity Intolerance
   Airway Clearance, Ineffective
   Breathing Patterns, Ineffective
   Cardiac Output, Alteration in: Decreased
   Diversional Activity Deficit
   Gas Exchange, Impaired
   Home Maintenance Management, Impaired
   Mobility, Impaired Physical
   † Respiratory Function, Potential Alteration in
   Self-care Deficit: (Total, Feeding, Bathing/Hygiene, Dressing/
      Grooming, Toileting)
   Tissue Perfusion, Alteration in: (Cerebral, Cardiopulmonary,
      Renal, Gastrointestinal, Peripheral)

5. Sleep–rest pattern
   Sleep Pattern Disturbance

6. Cognitive–perceptual pattern
   Comfort, Altered: Acute Pain
   Comfort, Altered: Chronic Pain
   Hyperthermia
   Hypothermia
   Knowledge Deficit: (specify)
   Sensory–Perceptual Alterations: (Visual, Auditory, Kines-
      thetic, Gustatory, Tactile, Olfactory)
   Thought Processes, Alteration in
   Unilateral Neglect

7. Self-perception pattern
   Anxiety
   Fear
   Hopelessness
   Powerlessness
   Self-concept, Disturbance in

8. Role–relationship pattern
   † Communication, Impaired

Communication, Impaired Verbal
Family Processes, Alteration in
Grieving: (specify)
Parenting, Alteration in
† Parental Role, Alteration in
Social Interaction, Impaired
Social Isolation

9. Sexuality–reproductive pattern
Sexual Dysfunction
Sexuality Patterns, Altered

10. Coping–stress tolerance pattern
Adjustment, Impaired
Coping, Ineffective Individual
Coping, Ineffective Family
Post-trauma Response
Rape Trauma Syndrome
† Self-harm, Potential for
Violence, Potential for

11. Value–belief pattern
Spiritual Distress

---

* The Functional Health Patterns were identified in Gordon M:
Nursing Diagnosis: Process and Application. New York,
McGraw-Hill, 1982, with minor changes by the author.

† These categories have been added by the author.

Acknowledgments

I would like to thank the following people for their consultation during the development of the manual:

Rosalinda Alfaro, R.N., M.S.N.
  Nursing Consultant
  Malvern, Pennsylvania

Cynthia Balin, R.N., M.S.N.
  Director of Clinical Services
  Kissimmee Memorial Hospital
  Kissimmee, Florida

Ann Curtis, R.N., B.S.N.
  Staff Development Department
  Wilmington Medical Center
  Wilmington, Delaware

Jacqueline W. Levett, R.N., M.S.N.
  Pediatric Clinical Specialist
  Wilmington Medical Center
  Wilmington, Delaware

Mary Sieggreen, M.S.N., R.N., C.S.
  Clinical Nurse Specialist
  Vascular Surgery
  Harper Hospital
  Detroit Medical Center
  Detroit, Michigan

Mary Mishler Vogel, R.N., M.S.N.
  Instructor
  Helene Fuld School of Nursing
  Camden, New Jersey

Anne E. Willard, R.N., M.S.N.
  Associate Professor
  Cumberland County College
  Vineland, New Jersey

A sincere "thank you" to my diligent typist, Maria Manel; and once again, to my husband, Richard, for his support on yet another project

Contents

Section II
MEDICAL DIAGNOSTIC CATEGORIES WITH ASSOCIATED NURSING DIAGNOSES AND COLLABORATIVE PROBLEMS   127

Medical Diagnoses   129

Pediatric/Adolescent Disorders **218**

Section I

Nursing Diagnostic Categories

Activity Intolerance

DEFINITION

Activity Intolerance: The state in which the individual experiences an inability, physiologically and psychologically, to endure or tolerate an increase in activity.

DEFINING CHARACTERISTICS

Major (Must Be Present)

Altered response to activity
  Respiratory
    Dyspnea
    Shortness of breath

    Excessive increase in
      rate
    Decrease in rate

  Pulse
    Weak
    Decrease in rate
    Excessive increase in
      rate
  Blood pressure
    Failure to increase
      with activity
    Increase in diastolic
      by 15 mm Hg
  Weakness
  Fatigue

    Failure to return to
      resting after
      three minutes
    Rhythm change

    Decrease

Minor (May Be Present)

  Pallor or cyanosis
  Confusion
  Vertigo

ETIOLOGICAL, CONTRIBUTING, RISK FACTORS

Any factor that causes fatigue or compromises oxygen transport can cause activity intolerance. Some common factors are listed below.

Pathophysiological

Alterations in the oxygen transport system
  Cardiac
    Congestive heart   Angina
      failure   Myocardial infarction
    Arrhythmias
  Respiratory
    Chronic obstructive pulmonary disease
  Circulatory
    Anemia
    Peripheral arterial disease
  Acute infection
    Viral infection
    Mononucleosis
    Hepatitis
  Chronic infection
    Endocarditis
    Tuberculosis
  Endocrine or metabolic disorders
    Diabetes mellitus
    Hypothyroidism
    Pituitary disorders
    Addison's disease
  Chronic diseases
    Renal   Musculoskeletal
    Hepatic   Neurological
  Nutritional disorders
    Obesity
    Malnourishment
    Inadequate diet
  Hypovolemia
  Electrolyte imbalance
  Malignancies

Treatment-related

Surgery
Diagnostic studies
Treatment schedule/treatments (frequency)
Prolonged bed rest
Medications
  Antihypertensives
  Minor tranquilizers
  Hypnotics

Antidepressants
Antihistamines

Situational (Personal, Environmental)

Depression
Lack of motivation
Sedentary life-style
Extreme stress
Crisis—personal or developmental, career, family,
      financial
Stressors (*e.g.*)
   Impaired language   Impaired motor
         function   function
   Impaired sensory   Pain
         function
Fatigue
   Caused by (*e.g.*)
      Sensory overload   Equipment that
      Sensory deprivation   requires strength
      Interrupted sleep   (walkers,
                                    crutches, braces)
                                 Gait disorders
                                 Stress

Maturational

Elderly (sensory-motor deficit)

Adjustment, Impaired*

DEFINITION

Impaired Adjustment: The state in which the individual is
unable to modify his/her life-style/behavior in a manner
consistent with a change in health status.

* Note: The term *adjustment* describes an individual's psychosocial regulatory processes to establish equilibrium in a person-
environment.

DEFINING CHARACTERISTICS

Major (Must Be Present)

Verbalization of nonacceptance of health status change or inability to be involved in problem solving or goal setting

Minor (May Be Present)

Lack of movement toward independence; extended period of shock, disbelief, or anger regarding health status change; lack of future-oriented thinking

ETIOLOGICAL, CONTRIBUTING, RISK FACTORS

Adjustment impairment can result from a variety of situations and health problems. Some common sources are listed below.

Pathophysiological

Spinal cord injury
Paralysis
Loss of limb
Cerebrovascular accident (CVA)
Myocardial infarction
Progressive neurological diseases
Cancer
Chronic obstructive pulmonary disease (COPD)

Treatment-related

Dialysis

Situational (Personal, Environmental)

Inadequate support systems
Unavailable support systems
Impaired cognition
Depression
Loss (object, person, job)
Divorce

Maturational

Child/adolescent: chronic disease, disability
Adult: loss of ability to practice vocation, role reversal
Elderly: normal physiological aging changes

Anxiety

DEFINITION

Anxiety: A state in which the individual experiences feelings of uneasiness (apprehension) and activation of the autonomic nervous system in response to a vague, nonspecific threat.*

DEFINING CHARACTERISTICS

Major (Must Be Present)

Manifested by symptoms from three categories—physiological, emotional, and cognitive. Symptoms vary according to the level of anxiety.

Physiological

Increased heart rate
Insomnia
Elevated blood pressure
Fatigue and weakness
Increased respiratory rate
Flushing or pallor
Diaphoresis
Dry mouth
Dilated pupils
Body aches and pains
    (especially chest,
    back, neck)

Voice tremors/pitch
    changes
Trembling
Restlessness
Palpitations
Faintness/dizziness
Nausea and/or vomiting
Paresthesias
Frequent urination
Hot and cold flashes
Diarrhea

Emotional

Person states that he has feelings of
Apprehension
Lack of self-confidence
Helplessness
Losing control
Nervousness
Tension, or being "keyed
    up"

Fear
Inability to relax
Unreality
Anticipation of
    misfortune

* Anxiety differs from fear in that the anxious person cannot identify the threat. With fear, the threat can be identified.

Person exhibits
  Irritability/impatience
  Criticism of self and others
  Angry outbursts
  Withdrawal
  Crying
  Lack of initiative
  Tendency to blame others
  Self-depreciation
  Startle reaction

Cognitive

  Inability to concentrate
  Lack of awareness of surroundings
  Forgetfulness
  Rumination
  Orientation to past rather than to present or future
  Blocking of thoughts (inability to remember)
  Hyperattentiveness

Etiological, Contributing, Risk Factors

Pathophysiological

  Any factor that interferes with the basic human needs
    for food, air, and comfort

Situational (Personal, Environmental)

Actual or perceived threat to self-concept
  Change in status and prestige
  Failure (or success)
  Lack of recognition from others
  Loss of valued possessions
  Ethical dilemmas

Actual or perceived loss of significant others
  Death
  Divorce
  Cultural pressures
  Moving
  Temporary or permanent separation

Actual or perceived threat to biological integrity
  Dying
  Assault
  Invasive procedures
  Disease

Actual or perceived change in environment
  Hospitalization
  Safety hazards

Moving   Environmental
Retirement   pollutants
Actual or perceived change in socioeconomic status
Unemployment   Promotion
New job
Transmission of another person's anxiety to the
individual

Maturational (Threat to Developmental Task)

Infant/child
Separation
Mutilation
Peer relationships
Achievement
Adolescent
Sexual development
Peer relationships
Independence
Adult
Pregnancy
Parenting
Career development
Effects of aging
Elderly
Sensory losses
Motor losses
Financial problems
Retirement

Body Temperature, Alteration in

Hypothermia

Hyperthermia

Thermoregulation, Ineffective

DEFINITION

Alteration in Body Temperature: The state in which the individual has failed or is at risk of failing to maintain body temperature within normal range because of internal factors.*

DEFINING CHARACTERISTICS

Major (Must Be Present)

Change in body temperature
Presence of risk factors (etiological, contributing factors)

ETIOLOGICAL, CONTRIBUTING, RISK FACTORS

Pathophysiological

Illness or trauma affecting temperature regulation:
Coma/increased intracranial pressure
Brain tumor/hypothalamic tumor/head trauma
Cerebrovascular accident (CVA)
Infection
Integument (skin) injury
Anemia
Neurovascular disease/peripheral vascular disease
Pheochromocytoma (tumor of the adrenal medulla)
Altered metabolic rate

* Note: These diagnostic categories represent two distinct thermal problems. One (Alteration in Body Temperature) is primarily caused by internal factors (*e.g.,* infection, disease), and the nurse does not treat the factors but focuses on comfort and hydration. The other two (Hypothermia, Hyperthermia) are caused by external factors (climate, nutrition), and the nurse focuses on helping the client adapt to or control these factors. An individual with the diagnosis of Hypothermia or Hyperthermia may be in a life-threatening situation that requires medical consultation. The nursing focus for Hyperthermia and Hypothermia is *prevention.* That is, *Potential* Hyperthermia or *Potential* Hypothermia would better describe the nursing role.

Treatment-related
Medications (*e.g.*, vasodilators/vasoconstrictors)
Sedation
Parenteral fluid infusion/blood transfusion
Dialysis
Surgery
Hypothermia/hyperthermia blanket

Maturational
Extremes of age (*e.g.*, newborn, elderly)

Hypothermia

DEFINITION

Hypothermia: The state in which an individual has or is at risk for a sustained reduction of body temperature of below 35°C (95°F) orally or 36°C (96°F) rectally.

DEFINING CHARACTERISTICS

Major (Must Be Present)

Reduction in body temperature below 35°C (95°F) orally or 36°C (96°F) rectally

Minor (May Be Present)

Cool skin
Pallor/blanching/redness of skin
Mental confusion/drowsiness/restlessness
Decreased pulse and respiration
Shivering
Cachexia/malnutrition

ETIOLOGICAL, CONTRIBUTING, RISK FACTORS

Situational (Personal, Environmental)

Exposure to heat, cold, sun, rain, snow, wind
Inappropriate clothing for climate
Poverty (inability to pay for shelter or heat)
Extremes of weight

Dehydration
Inactivity or vigorous activity
Exposure to communicable disease (*e.g.*, measles)

Maturational

Extremes of age (*e.g.*, newborn, elderly)

Hyperthermia

DEFINITION

Hyperthermia: The state in which an individual has or is at risk for a sustained elevation of body temperature of greater than 37.8°C. (100°F) orally or 38.8°C. (101°F) rectally due to external factors.

DEFINING CHARACTERISTICS

Major (Must Be Present)

Temperature greater than 37.8°C (100°F) orally or 38.8°C (101°F) rectally

Minor (May Be Present)

Flushed skin
Warm to touch
Increased respiratory rate
Tachycardia
Seizures/convulsions
Shivering/Goose pimples
Dehydration
Specific or generalized aches and pains (*e.g.*, headache)
Malaise/fatigue/weakness
Loss of appetite
Drowsiness/confusion/restlessness

ETIOLOGICAL, CONTRIBUTING, RISK FACTORS

Situational (Personal, Environmental)

Exposure to heat, cold, sun, rain, snow, wind
Inappropriate clothing for climate

Poverty
Extremes of weight
Dehydration
Inactivity or vigorous activity
Lack of knowledge

Maturational

Extremes of age (*e.g.*, newborn, elderly)

Thermoregulation, Ineffective*

DEFINITION

Ineffective Thermoregulation: The state in which an individual experiences or is at risk of experiencing an inability to effectively maintain normal body temperature in the presence of adverse or changing external factors.

DEFINING CHARACTERISTICS

Major (Must Be Present)

Temperature fluctuations related to limited metabolic compensatory regulation in response to environmental factors.

ETIOLOGICAL, CONTRIBUTING, RISK FACTORS

Situational (Personal, Environmental)

Fluctuating environmental temperatures
Cold or wet articles (clothes, cribs, equipment)
Inadequate heating system

* This diagnostic category is indicated when the nurse can maintain or assist an individual to maintain a body temperature within normal limits by manipulating external factors (*e.g.*, clothing) and environmental conditions. Individuals who are at high risk for this diagnosis are the elderly and neonates. For individuals with temperature fluctuations due to disease, infections, or trauma, see *Alteration in Body Temperature.*

Inadequate housing
Wet body surface
Inadequate clothing for weather (excessive, insufficient)

Maturational

Neonate
Large surface area relative to body mass
Limited ability to produce heat (metabolic)
Limited shivering ability
Increased basal metabolism
Premature (same as neonate but more severe)
Elderly
Decreased basal metabolism
Loss of adipose tissue (limbs)

Bowel Elimination, Alterations in: Constipation

DEFINITION

Constipation: The state in which the individual experiences or is at high risk of experiencing stasis of the large intestine, resulting in infrequent elimination and hard, dry feces.

DEFINING CHARACTERISTICS

Major (Must Be Present)

Hard, formed stool
Defecation occurs fewer than three times a week

Minor (May Be Present)

Decreased bowel sounds
Reported feeling of rectal fullness
Reported feeling of pressure in rectum
Straining and pain on defecation
Palpable impaction

ETIOLOGICAL, CONTRIBUTING, RISK FACTORS

Pathophysiological

Malnutrition
Sensory-motor disorders
  Spinal cord lesions
  Spinal cord injury
        Cerebrovascular
          accident (CVA,
          stroke)
        Neurological diseases
Metabolic and endocrine disorders
  Anorexia nervosa
  Obesity
        Hypothyroidism
        Hyperparathyroidism
Ileus
Pain (upon defecation)
  Hemorrhoids
  Back injury
Decreased peristalsis related to hypoxia (cardiac,
    pulmonary)
Megacolon

Treatment-related

Drug side-effects
  Antacids
  Iron
  Barium
  Aluminum
        Calcium
        Anticholinergics
        Anesthetics
        Narcotics (codeine,
          morphine)

Surgery
Habitual laxative use

Situational (Personal, Environmental)

Immobility
Pregnancy
Stress
Lack of exercise
Irregular evacuation
    patterns
        Lack of privacy
        Inadequate diet (lack of
          roughage/thiamine)
        Dehydration
        Fear of rectal or cardiac
          pain

Maturational

Infant
  Formula
Child
  Toilet training (reluctance to interrupt play)

Elderly
Decreased motility of gastrointestinal tract

Bowel Elimination, Alterations in: Diarrhea

DEFINITION

Diarrhea: The state in which the individual experiences or is at high risk of experiencing frequent passage of liquid stool or unformed stool.

DEFINING CHARACTERISTICS

Major (Must Be Present)
Loose, liquid stools
Increased frequency

Minor (May Be Present)
Urgency
Cramping/abdominal pain
Increased frequency of bowel sounds
Increase in fluidity or volume of stools

ETIOLOGICAL, CONTRIBUTING, RISK FACTORS

Pathophysiological

Nutritional disorders and malabsorptive syndromes
Kwashiorkor Crohn's disease
Gastritis Lactose intolerance
Peptic ulcer Spastic colon
Diverticulitis Celiac disease (sprue)
Ulcerative colitis Irritable bowel
Metabolic and endocrine disorders
Diabetes mellitus Thyrotoxicosis
Addison's disease
Dumping syndrome
Infectious process
Trichinosis Shigellosis

Dysentery
Cholera
Malaria
Cancer
Uremia
Tuberculosis
Arsenic poisoning
Fecal impaction

Typhoid fever
Infectious hepatitis

Treatment-related

Surgical intervention of the bowel
Loss of bowel   Ileal bypass
Drug side-effects
Thyroid agents   Stool softeners
Antacids   Antibiotics
Laxatives   Cancer
                                   chemotherapeutic
                                   agents

Tube feedings

Cardiac Output, Alterations In: Decreased (Specify)

DEFINITION

Alterations in Cardiac Output: Decreased: A state in which the individual experiences a reduction in the amount of blood pumped by the heart, resulting in compromised cardiac function.

DEFINING CHARACTERISTICS

Low blood pressure   Dysrhythmia
Rapid pulse   Oliguria
Restlessness   Fatigability
Cyanosis   Vertigo
Dyspnea   Edema (peripheral, sacral)
Angina

Note: This diagnostic category represents a situation in which nurses have multiple responsibilities. Individuals experiencing decreased cardiac output may present various responses that disrupt functioning, such as:

Activity intolerance

Sleep/rest dysrhythm

Or they may be at risk for developing physiological complications, such as:

Arrhythmias

Cardiogenic shock

Congestive heart failure

I recommend that the nurse not use *Alterations in Cardiac Output: Decreased* but instead select another diagnostic category that better describes the situation. (Refer to Activity Intolerance.)

It is also recommended that the physiological complications that nurses monitor for in individuals with decreased cardiac output, and for which they collaborate with medicine for treatment, be labeled collaborative problems, such as

Potential complication:

Arrhythmias

Cardiogenic shock

Hypoxia

By not using *Alteration in Cardiac Output: Decreased,* the nurse can more specifically describe the situations that nurses treat either as a nursing diagnosis or as a collaborative problem.

Comfort, Altered

Comfort, Altered: Acute Pain

Comfort, Altered: Chronic Pain

DEFINITION

Altered Comfort: A state in which the individual experiences an uncomfortable sensation in response to a noxious stimulus.

DEFINING CHARACTERISTICS

Major (Must Be Present)

The person reports or demonstrates a discomfort.

Minor (May Be Present)

Autonomic response in acute pain
    Blood pressure increased
    Pulse increased
    Respirations increased
    Diaphoresis
    Dilated pupils
Guarded position
Facial mask of pain
Crying, moaning

ETIOLOGICAL, CONTRIBUTING, RISK FACTORS

Any factor can contribute to altered comfort. The most common are listed below.

Pathophysiological

Musculoskeletal disorders
    Fractures   Arthritis
    Contractures   Spinal cord disorders
    Spasms
Visceral disorders
    Cardiac   Intestinal
    Renal   Pulmonary
Cancer
Vascular disorders
    Vasospasm   Phlebitis
    Occlusion   Vasodilation (headache)
Inflammation
    Nerve   Joint
    Tendon   Muscle
    Bursa
Contagious disease (rubella, chickenpox)

Treatment-related

Trauma (surgery, accidents)
    Diagnostic tests
        Venipuncture

> Invasive scanning (*e.g.,* intravenous pyelogram [IVP])
> Biopsy
Medications

Situational (Personal, Environmental)
Immobility/improper positioning
Overactivity
Pressure points (tight cast, Ace bandage)
Pregnancy (prenatal, intrapartum, postpartum)
Allergic response
Chemical irritants
Stress

Altered Comfort: Acute Pain

DEFINITION

Acute Pain: The state in which an individual experiences pain that can last from one second to as long as six months. It subsides with healing or when the stimulus is removed.

DEFINING CHARACTERISTICS

Major (Must Be Present)

The person reports or exhibits pain (may be the only sign of pain).

Minor (May Be Present)
Fear of pain
Inability to concentrate
Guarded positioning
Muscle spasm
Increase in pulse, blood pressure, and respiration
Evidence of inflammation (redness, heat, swelling)
Rubbing or pulling of body part
Tense body posture

Altered Comfort: Chronic Pain

DEFINITION

Chronic Pain: The state in which an individual experiences pain that is persistent or intermittent and lasts for more than six months.

DEFINING CHARACTERISTICS

Major (Must Be Present)

The person reports that pain has existed for more than six months (may be the only assessment data present).

Minor (May Be Present)

Discomfort
Anger, frustration, depression because of situation
Facial mask of pain
Anorexia, weight loss
Insomnia
Guarded movement
Muscle spasms
Redness, swelling, heat
Color changes in affected area
Reflex abnormalities

Communication, Impaired*

Communication, Impaired Verbal

DEFINITION

Impaired Communication: The state in which the individual experiences, or could experience, a decreased ability to send or receive messages (*i.e.,* has difficulty exchanging thoughts, ideas, or desires).

DEFINING CHARACTERISTICS

Major (Must Be Present)

Inappropriate or absent speech or response

* This diagnostic category represents communication problems that involve both sending and receiving messages (talking and listening).

Minor (May Be Present)

Stuttering
Slurring
Problem in finding the correct word when speaking
Weak or absent voice
Decreased auditory comprehension
Deafness or inattention to noises or voices
Confusion
Inability to speak dominant language

ETIOLOGICAL, CONTRIBUTING, RISK FACTORS

Pathophysiological

Cerebral impairment
  Expressive or receptive aphasia
  Cerebrovascular accident (CVA)
  Brain damage (*e.g.*, birth/head trauma
  Central nervous system (CNS) depression/increased
    intracranial pressure
  Tumor (head, neck, or spinal cord)
  Mental retardation
  Chronic hypoxia/decreased cerebral blood flow
Neurologic impairment
  Quadriplegia
  Nervous system diseases (*e.g.*, myasthenia gravis,
    multiple sclerosis)
  Vocal cord paralysis
  Auditory nerve damage
Respiratory impairment (*e.g.*, shortness of breath)
Auditory impairment (decreased hearing)
Laryngeal edema/infection

Treatment-Related

Surgery
  Endotracheal intubation
  Tracheostomy/tracheotomy/laryngectomy
  Surgery of the head, face, neck, or mouth
  Pain (especially of the mouth or throat)
  Drugs (*e.g.*, central nervous system [CNS]
    depressants, anesthesia)

Situational (Personal, Environmental)

Fatigue (affecting ability to listen)

No access to hearing aid/malfunction of hearing aid
Oral deformities
  Cleft lip or palate
  Malocclusion or fractured jaw
  Missing teeth
Speech pathology
  Stuttering
  Lisping
  Ankyloglossia ("tongue-tied")
  Voice problems
Language barrier (unfamiliar language or dialect)
Psychological barrier (*e.g.,* fear, shyness)
Lack of privacy
Lack of support system
Loss of recent memory recall

Maturational
  Elderly (auditory losses)
  Infants
  Children

Communication, Impaired Verbal

DEFINITION

Impaired Verbal Communication: The state in which the individual experiences, or could experience, a decreased ability or inability to speak but can understand others.

DEFINING CHARACTERISTICS

Major (Must Be Present)
  Inability to speak words but can understand others
  or
  Articulation or motor planning deficits

Minor (May Be Present)
  Shortness of breath

ETIOLOGICAL, CONTRIBUTIONS, RISK FACTORS

See *Impaired Communication.*

Coping, Ineffective Individual

DEFINITION

Ineffective Individual Coping: A state in which the individual experiences or is at risk of experiencing an inability to manage internal or environmental stressors adequately because of inadequate resources (physical, psychological, or behavioral).

DEFINING CHARACTERISTICS*

Major (Must Be Present)

Change in usual communication patterns
Verbalization of inability to cope
Inappropriate use of defense mechanisms
Inability to meet role expectations

Minor (May Be Present)

Anxiety
Reported life stress
Inability to problem-solve
Alteration in social participation
Destructive behavior toward self or others
High incidence of accidents
Frequent illnesses
Verbalization of inability to ask for help
Verbal manipulation
Inability to meet basic needs

ETIOLOGICAL, CONTRIBUTING, RISK FACTORS

Pathophysiological

Changes in body integrity
Loss of body part

* Adapted from Vincent KG: The validation of a nursing diagnosis. Nurs Clin North Am 20(4):631–639, 1985

Disfigurement secondary to trauma
Altered affect caused by changes in
  Body chemistry
  Tumor (brain)
  Intake of mood-altering substance
Physiological manifestations of
  Persistent stress

Situational (Personal, Environmental)

Changes in physical environment

War	Seasonal work (migrant
Natural disaster	worker)
Relocation	Poverty

Disruption of emotional bonds due to

Death	Relocation
Separation or divorce	Incarceration
Desertion	

Unsatisfactory support system
Institutionalization

Jail	Educational institution
Foster home	Maintenance institution
Orphanage	for the disabled

Sensory overload
  Factory environment
  Urbanization: crowding,
      noise pollution,
      excessive activity
Inadequate psychological resources

Poor self-esteem	Helplessness
Excessive negative	Lack of motivation to
beliefs about self	respond

Culturally related conflicts with life

Experiences	Abortion
Premarital sex	

Maturational

Child

Developmental tasks	Competition among
(independence vs.	peers
dependence)	Peer relationships
Entry into school	

Adolescent

Physical and emotional	Sexual awareness
changes	Educational demands

Independence from
family
Heterosexual
relationships

Career choices

Young adult
Career choices
Educational demands
Leaving home

Marriage
Parenthood

Middle adult
Physical signs of aging
Career pressures
Child-rearing problems

Problems with relatives
Social status needs
Aging parents

Elderly
Physical changes
Changes in financial
status
Changes in residence

Retirement
Response of others to
older people

Treatment-related

Separation from family and home (*e.g.,* hospitalizaton,
confinement to a nursing home)
Need for medical treatment conflicts with beliefs (*e.g.,*
Christian Scientist)
Disfigurement due to surgery
Alteration in appearance due to drugs, radiation, or
other treatment
Altered affect due to hormonal therapy
Sensory overload due to medical technology (*e.g.,*
critical care units)

Coping, Ineffective Family

DEFINITION

Ineffective Family Coping: The state in which a family
demonstrates destructive behavior in response to an inability

to manage internal or external stressors due to inadequate resources (physical, psychological, cognitive, and/or behavioral).*

DEFINING CHARACTERISTICS

Since disturbances in family coping can be manifested in a variety of ways, there is no typical response. All do reflect a lack of mutual need attainment within the family. Reactions may include the following:

Neglectful care of the client in regard to basic human needs and/or illness-related treatments

Neglect of other family members (abandonment, desertion)

Distortion of reality regarding the client's health problem, including prolonged denial

Unresolved emotions of anger, depression, hostility, and aggression

Verbalization of abuse by spouse

Child abuse

Helpless, inactive dependency of client

Marital/parental conflict

Behavior problems in children

Etiological, Contributing, Risk Factors

The following describes those individuals or families who are at high risk for contributing to a family's destructive coping behavior.

Parent(s)

Single	Drug addicted
Adolescent	Terminally ill
Abusive	Acute disability/
Emotionally disturbed	accident
Alcoholic	Elderly dependent

* The nursing diagnosis *Ineffective Family Coping* describes a family that has a history of demonstrating destructive behavior. This diagnosis differs from *Alteration in Family Processes,* which describes a family that usually functions constructively but is challenged by a stressor that has altered or may alter its function.

Child
Of unwanted pregnancy
Of undesired sex
With undesired
    characteristics
Physically handicapped

Mentally handicapped
Hyperactive
Terminally ill
Adolescent rebellion

Situational
Separation from
    nuclear family
Lack of extended
    family
Lack of knowledge
Economic problems
    (inflation,
    unemployment)
Change in family unit
    (*e.g.,* new child,
    relative moves in)
Relationship problems

Marital discord
Divorce
Separation
Step-parents
Live-in sexual partner
Relocation

Other
History of ineffective relationship with own parents
History of abusive relationships with parents
Unrealistic expectations of child by parent
Unrealistic expectations of self by parent
Unrealistic expectations of parent by child
Unmet psychosocial needs of child by parent
Unmet psychosocial needs of parent by child

Diversional Activity Deficit

DEFINITION

Diversional Activity Deficit: The state in which the individual experiences or is at risk of experiencing an environment that is devoid of stimulation or interest.

DEFINING CHARACTERISTICS

Major (Must Be Present)
  Statements of boredom/depression from inactivity

Minor (May Be Present)
  Constant expression of unpleasant thoughts or feelings
  Yawning or inattentiveness
  Flat facial expression
  Body language (shifting of body away from speaker)
  Restlessness/fidgeting
  Immobile (on bed rest or confined)
  Weight loss or gain
  Hostility

ETIOLOGICAL, CONTRIBUTING, RISK FACTORS

Pathophysiological
  Communicable disease
  Pain

Treatment-related
  Long or frequent treatments

Situational (Personal, Environmental)
  No peers or friends
  Monotonous environment
  Long-term hospitalization or confinement
  Lack of motivation
  Loss of ability to perform usual or favorite activities
  Excessive long hours of stressful work
  No time for leisure activities
  Career changes (*e.g.,* teacher to homemaker, retirement)
  Children leaving home ("empty nest")
  Immobility
  Decreased sensory perception (*e.g.,* blindness, hearing
    loss)

Maturational
  Infants/children
    Lack of appropriate toys/peers

Elderly
  Sensory-motor deficits

Family Processes, Alterations in

DEFINITION

Alterations in Family Processes: The state in which a normally supportive family experiences a stressor that challenges its previously effective functioning ability.*

DEFINING CHARACTERISTICS

Major (Must Be Present)

Family system cannot or does not
  Adapt constructively to crisis
  Communicate openly and effectively between family members

Minor (May Be Present)

Family system cannot or does not
  Meet physical needs of all its members
  Meet emotional needs of all its members
  Meet spiritual needs of all its members
  Express or accept a wide range of feelings
  Seek or accept help appropriately

ETIOLOGICAL, CONTRIBUTING, RISK FACTORS

Any factor can contribute to an alteration in family processes. Some common factors are listed below.

* The nursing diagnosis *Alterations in Family Processes* describes a family that usually functions optimally but is challenged by a stressor that has altered or may alter the family's function. This diagnosis differs from *Ineffective Family Coping,* which describes a family that has a pattern of destructive behavioral responses.

Pathophysiological
Illness of family member
  Discomforts related to
      the symptoms of
      the illness
  Change in the family
      member's ability
      to function
  Time-consuming
      treatments
Trauma
  Surgery

Disabling treatments
Expensive treatments

Loss of body part or
    function

Treatment-related
Disruption of family routines due to time-consuming
    treatments (*e.g.*, home dialysis)
Physical changes due to treatments of ill family
    member
Emotional changes in all family members due to
    treatments of ill family member
Financial burden of treatments for ill family member
Hospitalization of ill family member

Situational (Personal, Environmental)
Loss of family member
  Death
  Going away to school
  Separation
  Divorce
Gain of new family member
  Birth
  Adoption
Poverty
Disaster
Relocation
Economic crisis
  Unemployment
Change in family roles
  Working mother
Birth of child with defect

Incarceration
Desertion
Hospitalization

Marriage
Elderly relative

Financial loss

Retirement

Conflict
    Goal conflicts
    Moral conflict with
       reality
    Cultural conflict with
       reality
    Personality conflict in
       family

Breach of trust between members
    Dishonesty
    Adultery
History of psychiatric illness in family
Social deviance by family member (including crime)

Fear

DEFINITION

Fear: A state in which the individual experiences a feeling of physiological or emotional disruption related to an identifiable source that the person perceives as dangerous.*

DEFINING CHARACTERISTICS

Major (Must Be Present)

Feelings of: dread, fright, apprehension
Behaviors of: avoidance, narrowing of focus on danger, and deficits in attention, performance, and control

Minor (May Be Present)

Verbal reports of: panic, obsessions
Behavioral acts of
    Aggression
    Escape
    Hypervigilance

---

* Fear differs from anxiety in that the person can identify the threat, while in anxiety the threat cannot be accurately identified. Although it is possible for fear to be present without anxiety, fear and anxiety usually coexist clinically.

Dysfunctional immobility
Compulsive mannerisms
Increased questioning/verbalization
Visceral–somatic activity
  Musculoskeletal
    Muscle tightness
    Fatigue
  Cardiovascular
    Palpitations
    Rapid pulse
    Increased blood pressure
  Respiratory
    Shortness of breath
    Increase rate
  Gastrointestinal
    Anorexia
    Nausea/vomiting
    Diarrhea
  Genitourinary
    Urinary frequency
  Skin
    Flush/pallor
    Sweating
    Paresthesia
  Central nervous system (CNS)/perceptual
    Syncope
    Insomnia
    Lack of concentration
    Irritability
    Absentmindedness
    Nightmares
    Dilated pupils

ETIOLOGICAL, CONTRIBUTING, RISK FACTORS

Fear can occur as a response to a variety of health problems, situations, or conflicts. Some common sources are indicated below.

Pathophysiological

Loss of body part
Loss of body function
Disabling illness

Long-term disability
Terminal disease

Treatment-related

Hospitalization
Surgery and its outcome   Invasive procedures
Anesthesia   Lack of knowledge

Situational (Personal, Environmental)

Influences of others   Change or loss of
Pain   significant other
New environment   Divorce
New people   Success
Lack of knowledge   Failure

Maturational

Children
   Age-related fears (dark, strangers)
   Influence of others
Adolescent
   School adjustments,
   Social and intellectual competitiveness
   Independence
   Authorities
Adult
   Marriage
   Pregnancy
   Parenthood
Elderly
   Retirement
   Relinquishing roles
   Functional losses

Fluid Volume Deficit

DEFINITION

Fluid volume deficit: The state in which the individual experiences or is at risk of experiencing vascular, interstitial, or intracellular dehydration.

Note: This diagnostic category represents situations in which nurses can prescribe definitive treatment to prevent fluid depletion or to reduce or eliminate contributing factors such as insufficient oral intake. Situations that represent hypovolemia caused by hemorrhage or NPO states should be considered collaborative problems, not nursing diagnoses. Nurses monitor to detect these situations and collaborate with physicians for treatment. These situations can be labeled as *Potential complication: Hemorrhage,* or *Potential complication: Hypovolemia.*

DEFINING CHARACTERISTICS

Major (Must Be Present)

Output greater than intake
Increased serum sodium
Dry skin/mucous membranes

Minor (May Be Present)

Increased pulse rate (from baseline)
Decreased urine output or excessive urine output
Concentrated urine or urinary frequency
Decreased fluid intake
Weight loss (rapid)
Decreased venous filling
Hemoconcentration
Decreased pulse volume/pressure
Increased body temperature
Decreased skin turgor
Thirst/nausea/anorexia
Weakness/lethargy/confusion

ETIOLOGICAL, CONTRIBUTING, RISK FACTORS

Pathophysiological

Excessive urinary output
Uncontrolled diabetes
Diabetes insipidus (inappropriate antidiuretic hormone)
Burns
Fever or increased metabolic rate
Infection
Abnormal drainage
Wound

Excessive menses
Other
Serum electrolyte imbalance
Acid–base imbalance (acidosis–alkalosis)
Eclampsia (albumin loss)
Peritonitis
Diarrhea
Increased intracranial pressure

Treatment-related

Nasogastric suctioning
Imposed fluid restrictions
Preoperative period
Intraoperative period
Postoperative period

Situational (Personal, Environmental)

Vomiting/nausea
Decreased motivation to drink liquids
Depression
Fatigue
Dietary problems
Fad diets/fasting
Anorexia
High-solute tube feedings
Difficulty swallowing or feeding self
Oral pain
Fatigue
Climate exposure
Extreme heat/sun
Extreme dryness
Hyperpnea
Extreme exercise effort/diaphoresis
Excessive use of
Laxatives or enemas
Diuretics or alcohol

Maturational

Infant/child
Decreased fluid reserve
Decreased ability to concentrate urine
Elderly
Decreased fluid reserve
decreased sensation of thirst

Fluid Volume Excess*

DEFINITION

Fluid Volume Excess: The state in which the individual experiences or is at risk of experiencing intracellular or interstitial fluid overload.

DEFINING CHARACTERISTICS

Major (Must Be Present)

Edema

Taut, shiny skin

ETIOLOGICAL, CONTRIBUTING, RISK FACTORS

Pathophysiological

Renal failure, acute or chronic

Decreased cardiac output

Myocardial infarction   Valvular disease

Congestive heart failure   Tachycardia/

Left ventricular failure   arrhythmias

Varicosities of the legs

Liver disease

Cirrhosis   Cancer

Ascites

Tissue insult

Injury to the cell wall   Hypoxia of the cell

Inflammatory process

* This diagnostic category represents situations in which nurses can prescribe definitive treatment to reduce or eliminate factors that contribute to edema or can teach preventive actions. Situations that represent vascular fluid overload should be considered collaborative problems, not nursing diagnoses. They can be labeled *Potential complication: Congestive heart failure,* or *Potential complication: Hypervolemia*

Hormonal disturbances
   Pituitary   Estrogen
   Adrenal
Effusion (abnormal fluid accumulation)
   Pleural   Pericardial

Treatment-related

Corticosteroid therapy

Situational (Personal, Environmental)

Excessive sodium intake/fluid intake
Low protein intake
   Fad diets   Malnutrition
Dependent venous pooling/venostasis
   Immobility   Standing or sitting for
                              long periods
Venous pressure point
   Tight cast or bandage
Pregnancy
Inadequate lymphatic drainage

Maturational

Elderly (decreased cardiac output)

Grieving

DEFINITION

Grieving: A state in which an individual or family experiences an actual or perceived loss (person, object, function, status, relationship) or the state in which an individual or family responds to the realization of a future loss (anticipatory grieving).

DEFINING CHARACTERISTICS

Major (Must Be Present)

The person
   Reports an actual or perceived loss (person, object, function, status relationship)

or
Anticipates a loss

Minor (May Be Present)

Denial
Guilt
Anger
Despair
Feelings of worthlessness
Suicidal thoughts
Crying
Sorrow

Hallucinations
Delusions
Phobias
Anergia
Increased illnesses
Inability to concentrate
Visual, auditory, and
tactile hallucinations
about the object or
person

ETIOLOGICAL, CONTRIBUTING, RISK FACTORS

Pathophysiological

Loss of function (actual or potential) related to a body-system alteration

Neurological
Cardiovascular
Sensory
Musculoskeletal

Digestive
Respiratory
Renal

Loss of function or body part related to
Trauma

Treatment-related

Dialysis
Surgery (mastectomy, colostomy, hysterectomy)

Situational (Personal, Environmental)

Chronic pain
Terminal illness
Changes in life-style

Childbirth
Marriage
Separation

Divorce
Child leaving home
(*e.g.,* college or
marriage)
Loss of career

Type of relationship (with the person who is leaving or
is gone)
Multiple losses or crises
Lack of social support system

Maturational

Loss associated with aging

Friends
Occupation

Function
Home

Growth and Development, Altered*

DEFINITION

Altered Growth and Development: The state in which an individual has or is at risk for an impaired ability to perform tasks of his/her age group.

DEFINING CHARACTERISTICS

Major (Must Be Present)

Inability to perform or difficulty performing skills or behaviors typical of his/her age group; for example, motor, personal/social, language/cognition

Altered physical growth: Weight lagging behind height by two standard deviations; pattern of height and weight percentiles indicating a drop in pattern

Minor (May Be Present)

Inability to perform self-care or self-control activities appropriate for age

Flat affect, listlessness, decreased responses, slow in social responses, shows limited signs of satisfaction to caregiver, shows limited eye contact, difficulty feeding, decreased appetite, lethargic, irritable,

* The focus of this category will be children and adolescents. When an adult has not accomplished a developmental task, the nurse should assess for the altered functioning that has resulted from the failure to meet a developmental task; for example, Impaired Social Interactions or Ineffective Individual Coping.

negative mood, regression in self-toileting,
regression in self-feeding
Infants: watchfulness, interrupted sleep pattern

ETIOLOGICAL, CONTRIBUTING, RISK FACTORS

Pathophysiological

Circulatory impairment
  Congenital heart defects
  Congestive heart failure
Neurological impairment
  Cerebral damage
  Congenital defects
  Cerebral palsy
  Microcephaly
Gastrointestinal impairment
  Malabsorption syndrome
  Gastroesophageal reflux
  Cystic fibrosis
Endocrine or renal impairment
  Hormonal disturbance
Musculoskeletal impairments
  Congenital anomalies of extremities
  Muscular dystrophy
Acute illness
Prolonged pain
Repeated acute illness, chronic illness
Inadequate caloric, nutritional intake

Treatment-related

Prolonged, painful treatments
Repeated or prolonged hospitalization
Traction or casts that alter locomotion
Prolonged bed rest
Isolation due to disease processes
Confinement for ongoing treatment

Situational (Personal, Environmental)

Parental knowledge deficit
Stress (acute, transient, or chronic)
Hospitalization or change in usual environment

Separation from significant others (parents, primary
caregiver, or parents)
Inadequate, inappropriate parental support (neglect,
abuse)
Inadequate sensory stimulation (neglect, isolation)
Parent–child conflict
School-related stressors
Maternal or parental anxiety
Loss of significant other
Loss of control over environment (established rituals,
activities, established hours of contact with family)
Multiple caregivers

Maturational

Infant–Toddler

Lack of stimulation
Birth to three years
Separation from parents/significant others
Change in environment
Restriction of activity
Inadequate parental support
Inability to trust significant other
Inability to communicate (deafness)

Pre–school Age

Restriction of activity
Four to six years
Loss of ability to communicate
Lack of stimulation
Lack of significant other
Loss of significant other (death, divorce)
Loss of peer group
Loss of independence
Fear of mutilation/pain/abandonment
Removal from home environment

School Age

Loss of individual control
Six to eleven years
Loss of significant others
Loss of peer group
Fear of immobility, mutilation, death
Fear of intrusive procedures
Strange environment

Adolescent
Twelve to eighteen years
    Loss of independence and autonomy
    Disruption of peer relationships
    Disruption in body image
    Interruption of intellectual achievement
    Loss of significant other

Health Maintenance*

Health Maintenance, Alterations in

DEFINITION

Health Maintenance: The state in which the individual is at risk of experiencing a disruption in his present state of wellness because of inadequate knowledge of primary and secondary prevention or is assisted to a more healthful life-style.

* This diagnostic category can be used to describe the individual/ family that needs health teaching related to the promotion and maintenance of health (preventive behavior, age-related screening, optimal nutrition, etc.) The *Knowledge Deficit* diagnostic category describes the individual/family who needs teaching related to disease, disease management, and treatment.

This diagnostic category should be used to describe an asymptomatic person. However, it can be used for a person with a chronic disease to help that person attain a higher level of wellness. For example, a woman with lupus erythematosus can have the diagnosis *Health Maintenance: Lack of a regular exercise program.* This diagnostic category can also be used for persons with acute conditions to describe other dimensions of their health. For example, a child with acute otitis media may have the diagnosis *Health Maintenance: Bicycle safety* because he relates a lack of knowledge of safety measures for bicycles.

DEFINING CHARACTERISTICS

Major (Must Be Present)

Verbalizes a deficiency in knowledge
For health promotion
For health maintenance

ETIOLOGICAL, CONTRIBUTING, RISK FACTORS

Situational (Personal, Environmental)

Role changes
Marriage
Parenthood
"Empty-nest syndrome"
Retirement
Lack of knowledge of need for
Preventive behavior (disease)
Screening practices for age and risk
Optimal nutrition and weight control
Regular exercise program
Constructive stress management
Supportive social networks
Responsible role participation

Maturational

See table, Primary and Secondary Prevention for Age-related Situations, which follows.

Health Maintenance, Alterations in*

DEFINITION

Alterations in Health Maintenance: The state in which the individual experiences or is at risk of experiencing a disruption in his present state of wellness because of an unhealthy life-style.

* *Alteration in Health Maintenance* is a diagnostic category that describes a person who sustains an unhealthy life-style (obesity, tobacco use, frequent infections).

(*Text continues on p 52.*)

Primary and Secondary Prevention for Age-related Conditions

Developmental Level	Primary Prevention	Secondary Prevention

Infancy (0–1 year)	Parent education
	Infant safety
	Nutrition
	Breastfeeding
	Sensory stimulation
	Infant massage and touch
	Visual stimulation
	  Activity
	  Colors
	Auditory stimulation
	  Verbal
	  Music
	Immunizations
	DPT ⎫
	TOPV ⎭ at 2, 4, and 6 months
	Oral hygiene
	  Teething biscuits
	  Fluoride
	  Avoid sugared food and drink
		Complete physical examination every 2–3 months
		Screening at birth
		  Congenital hip
		  PKV
		  Sickel cell disease
		  Cystic fibrosis
		  Vision (startle reflex)
		  Hearing (response to and localization of sounds)
		Tuberculin test at 12 months
		Developmental assessments
		Screen and intervene for high risk
		  Low birth weight
		  Maternal substance abuse during pregnancy
		  Alcohol: fetal alcohol syndrome
		  Cigarettes: sudden infant death syndrome (SIDS)
		  Drugs: addicted neonate
		  Maternal infections during pregnancy

Primary and Secondary Prevention for Age-related Conditions (Continued)

Developmental Level	Primary Prevention	Secondary Prevention

Preschool (1–5 years)	Parent education
	  Teething
	  Discipline
	  Nutrition
	  Accident prevention
	  Normal growth and development
	Child education
	  Dental self-care
	  Dressing
	  Bathing with assistance
	  Feeding self-care
	Immunizations
	  DPT } at 18 months
	  TOPV }
	
	  MMR at 15 months
	Dental/oral hygiene
	  Fluoride treatments
	  Fluoridated water
	  Dietary counsel
		Complete physical exam between 2 and 3 years and preschool (U/A, CBC)
		Tuberculin test at 3 years
		Developmental assessments (annual)
		  Speech development
		  Hearing
		  Vision
		Screen and intervene
		  Plumbism
		  Developmental lag
		  Neglect or abuse
		  Strabismus
		  Hearing deficit
		  Vision deficit

**School age
(6–11 years)**

Health education of child
"Basic 4" nutrition
Accident prevention
Outdoor safety
Substance abuse counsel
Anticipatory guidance for physical
changes at puberty
Immunizations
Tetanus, age 10
DPT ⎫ boosters between
TOPV ⎭ 4 and 6 years
Dental hygiene every 6–12 months
Continue fluoridation
Complete physical examination

Complete physical examination
Tuberculin test every 3 years (at ages 6 and 9)
Developmental assessments
Language
Vision: Snellen charts at school
6–8 years, use "E" chart
Over 8 years, use alphabet chart
Hearing: audiogram

**Adolescence
(12–19 years)**

Health education
Proper nutrition and healthful diets
Sex education with family planning,
male/female
Safe driving skills
Adult challenges
Seeking employment and career
choices

Complete physical examination (prepuberty or
age 13)
Blood pressure
Cholesterol
Tuberculin test at 12 years
VDRL, CBC, U/A
Female: breast self-examination
Male: testicular self-examination

Primary and Secondary Prevention for Age-related Conditions (Continued)

Developmental Level	Primary Prevention	Secondary Prevention
	Dating and marriage Confrontation with substance abuse Safety in athletics Skin care Dental hygiene every 6–12 months Immunization Tetanus without trauma TOPV booster at 12–14 years	Female, if sexually active: Papanicolaou test and pelvic examination twice, one year apart (cervical gonorrhea culture with pelvic); then every 3 years if both are negative Screening and interventions if high risk Depression Suicide Substance abuse Pregnancy Family history of alcoholism or domestic violence
Young adult (20–39 years)	Health education Weight management with good nutrition as basal metabolic rate changes Life-style counseling Stress management skills	Complete physical examination at about 20 years, then every 5–6 years Cancer checkup every 3 years Female: breast self-examination monthly Male: testicular self-examination monthly

All females: baseline mammography between ages 35 and 40

Parents-to-be: high-risk screening for Down syndrome, Tay-Sachs disease

Pregnant female: screen for sexually transmitted disease, rubella titer, Rh factor

Screening and interventions if high risk

Female with previous breast cancer: annual mammography at 35 years and after

Female with mother or sister who has had breast cancer, same as above

Family history colorectal cancer or high risk: annual stool guaiac, digital rectal examination, and sigmoidoscopy

PPD if exposed to tuberculosis

Complete physical exam every 5–6 years with complete laboratory evaluation (serum/urine tests, x-ray, ECG)

Cancer checkup every year

Female: breast self-examination monthly

Male: testicular self-examination monthly

Safe driving
Family planning
Parenting skills
Regular exercise
Environmental health choices
Dental hygiene every 6–12 months
Immunization
Tetanus at 20 years and every 10 years
Female: rubella, if zero negative for antibodies

Health education: continue with young adult

Midlife changes, male and female counseling

"Empty-nest syndrome"

Anticipatory guidance for retirement

Grandparenting

Middle-aged adult (40–59 years)

Primary and Secondary Prevention for Age-related Conditions (Continued)

Developmental Level	Primary Prevention	Secondary Prevention
	Dental hygiene every 6–12 months	All females: annual mammography 50 years and over
	Immunizations	Schiøtz tonometry (glaucoma) every 3–5 years
	Tetanus every 10 years	Pregnant female: perinatal screening by amniocentesis if desired
	Pneumococcal } Annual if high risk; i.e., major chronic disease (COPD, CAD)	Sigmoidoscopy at 50 and 51, then every 4 years if negative
	Influenza	Stool guaiac annually at 50 and thereafter
		Screening and intervention if high risk
		Endometrial cancer: have endometrial sampling at menopause
		Oral cancer: screen more often if substance abuser
Elderly adult (60–74 years)	Health education: continue with previous counseling	Complete physical examination every 2 years with laboratory assessments
	Home safety	Annual cancer checkup
	Retirement	Blood pressure annually
	Loss of spouse	

Special health needs:
  Nutritional changes
  Changes in hearing or vision
  Alterations in bowel or bladder habits
  Dental/oral hygiene every 6–12 months
Immunizations
  Tetanus every 10 years
  Pneumococcal ⎱ annual if high risk
  Influenza   ⎰

Female: breast self-examination monthly
Male: testicular self-examination monthly
Female: annual mammogram
Annual stool guaiac
Sigmoidoscopy every 4 years
Schiøtz tonometry every 3–5 years
Podiatric evaluation with foot care PRN
Screen for high risk
  Depression
  Suicide

Old-age adult (75 years and over)

Health education: continue counsel
Anticipatory guidance
  Dying and death
  Loss of spouse
  Increasing dependency on others
Dental/oral hygiene every 6–12 months
Immunizations
  Tetanus every 10 years
  Pneumococcal ⎱ annual
  Influenza   ⎰

Complete physical exam annually
Laboratory assessments
Cancer checkup
Blood pressure
Stool guaiac
Female: mammogram, sigmoidoscopy every 4 years
Schiøtz tonometry every 3–5 years
Podiatrist PRN

DEFINING CHARACTERISTICS (in the Absence of Disease)

Major (Must Be Present)

Reports or demonstrates an unhealthy practice or life-style

Reports or demonstrates

Skin and nails

Malodorous	Sunburn
Unclean	Unusual color, pallor
Skin lesions (pustules, rashes, dry or scaly skin)	Unexplained scars

Respiratory system

Frequent infections	Dyspnea with exertion
Chronic cough	

Oral cavity

Frequent sores (on tongue, buccal mucosa)	Lesions associated with lack of oral care or substance abuse (leukoplakia, fistulas)
Loss of teeth at early age	

Gastrointestinal system and nutrition

Obesity	Chronic anemia
Anorexia	Chronic bowel irregularity
Cachexia	Chronic dyspepsia

Musculoskeletal system

Frequent muscle strain, backaches, neck pain

Diminished flexibility and muscle strength

Genitourinary system

Frequent venereal lesions and infections

Frequent use of potentially unhealthful over-the-counter products (chemical douches, perfumed vaginal products, nasal sprays, etc.)

Constitutional

Chronic fatigue, malaise, apathy

Neurosensory

Presence of facial tics (nonconvulsant)

Headaches

Psychoemotional

Emotional fragility

Behavior disorders (compulsiveness, belligerence)
Frequent feelings of being overwhelmed

ETIOLOGICAL, CONTRIBUTING, RISK FACTORS

Pathophysiological

Not directly related to Alterations in Health
Maintenance

Situational (Personal, Environmental)

Loss of independence
Changing support systems
Change in finances
Lack of knowledge
Poor learning skills
Crisis situation
Lack of access to adequate health care services
Substance abuse (alcohol, tobacco)
Inadequate health practice
Lack of supervision for dependents (children, elderly)
Health beliefs (lack of perceived threat to health)
Religious beliefs
External locus of control
Cultural or folk beliefs
Alterations in self-image (poor self-esteem, distorted
body image)

Maturational

Failure to practice age-related preventive measures
See table for age-related conditions.

Home Maintenance Management, Impaired

DEFINITION

Impaired Home Maintenance Management: The state in
which an individual or family experiences or is at risk of

experiencing a difficulty in maintaining self or family in a safe home environment.

DEFINING CHARACTERISTICS

Major (Must Be Present)

Outward expressions of difficulty by individual or family in maintaining the home (cleaning, repairs, financial needs)

or

In caring for self or family member at home

Minor (May Be Present)

Poor hygienic practices
  Infections
  Infestations
  Accumulated wastes
Impaired caregiver
  Overtaxed
  Anxious

Unwashed cooking and eating equipment
Offensive odors

Lack of knowledge
Negative response to ill member

Unavailable support system

ETIOLOGICAL, CONTRIBUTING, RISK FACTORS

Pathophysiological

Chronic debilitating disease
  Diabetes mellitus
  Chronic obstructive pulmonary disease
  Congestive heart failure
  Cancer

Arthritis
Multiple sclerosis
Muscular dystrophy

Situational (Personal, Environmental)

Injury to individual or family member (fractured limb, spinal cord injury)
Surgery (amputation, ostomy)
Impaired mental status (memory lapses, depression, anxiety—severe, panic)
Substance abuse (alcohol, other drugs)
Unavailable support system

Loss of family member
Addition of family member (newborn, aged parent)
Lack of knowledge
Insufficient finances

Maturational

Infant
  Newborn care
  High risk for sudden infant death syndrome
Elderly
  Family member with deficits (cognitive, motor,
    sensory)

Hopelessness*

DEFINITION

Hopelessness: A sustained subjective emotional state in which an individual sees no alternatives or personal choices available to solve problems or to achieve what is desired and cannot mobilize energy on own behalf to establish goals.

DEFINING CHARACTERISTICS

Major (Must Be Present)

Expresses profound, overwhelming apathy in response to a situation perceived as impossible with no solutions

Examples of expressions are

"I might as well give up because I can't make things better."

* Note: Hopelessness differs from powerlessness in that a hopeless person sees no solution to his problem and/or way to achieve what is desired, even if he/she has control of his/her life. A powerless person may see an alternative or answer to the problem yet be unable to do anything about it because of perceived lack of control and resources.

"My future seems awful to me."

"I can't imagine what my life will be like in ten years."

"I've never been given a break, so why should I in the future?"

"Life looks unpleasant when I think ahead."

"I know I'll never get what I really want."

"Things never work out how I want them to."

"It's foolish to want or get anything because I never do."

"It's unlikely that I'll get satisfaction in the future."

"The future seems vague and uncertain."

Physiological

Slowed responses to stimuli

Emotional

The hopeless person often has difficulty experiencing feelings, but may feel

Unable to seek good fortune, luck, or God's favor

That he/she has no meaning or purpose in life

"Empty or drained"

A sense of loss and deprivation

Person Exhibits

Passiveness

Decreased verbalization

Lack of ambition, initiative, and interest

Cognitive

Decreased problem-solving and decision-making capabilities

Deals with past and future, not the here and now

Decreased flexibility in thought processes

Lacks imagination and wishing capabilities

Unable to identify and/or accomplish desired objectives and goals

Unable to plan, organize, or make decisions

Unable to recognize sources of hope

Minor (May Be Present)

Physiological

Anorexia

Weight loss

Decreased exercise
Increased sleep

Emotional

Patient feels
Incompetent
"A lump in the throat"
Discouraged with self and others
"At the end of his/her rope"
Tense
Helpless
Overwhelmed ("I just can't . . .")
Loss of gratification from roles and relationships
Vulnerable

Person Exhibits

Poor eye contact; turns away from speaker; shrugs in
response to speaker
Apathy (decreased response to internal and external
stimuli)
Decreased affect
Decreased motivation
Despondency
Sighing
Social withdrawal
Lack of involvement in self-care (may be cooperative in
nursing care but offers little help to self)
Passively *allows* care
Regression
Resignation
Depression
Anger
Destructiveness

Cognitive

Conveys negative and/or slowed thought processes
Decreased ability to integrate information received
Loss of time perception for past, present, and future
Decreased ability to recall from the past
Confusion
Inability to communicate effectively
Distorted thought perceptions and associations
Unreasonable judgment
Suicidal thoughts
Unrealistic perceptions in relation to hope

ETIOLOGICAL, CONTRIBUTING, RISK FACTORS

Pathophysiological

Any chronic and/or terminal illness can cause or contribute to hopelessness (heart disease, kidney disease, cancer, acquired immune deficiency syndrome [AIDS]).
Associated risk factors include

Failing or deteriorating physiological condition

Impaired body image

New and unexpected signs or symptoms of previous disease process

Prolonged pain, discomfort, weakness

Impaired functional abilities (walking, elimination, eating)

Treatment-related

Prolonged treatments (*e.g.,* chemotherapy, radiation) that cause discomfort

Prolonged treatments with no positive results

Treatments that alter body image (*e.g.,* surgery, chemotherapy)

Prolonged diagnostic studies with no results

Prolonged dependence on equipment for life support (dialysis, respirator)

Prolonged dependence on equipment for monitoring bodily functions (telemetry)

Prolonged activity restriction (*e.g.,* fractures, spinal cord injury)

Prolonged isolation for disease processes (*e.g.,* infectious diseases, reverse isolation for suppressed immune system)

Situational (Personal, Environmental)

Separation from significant others (parents, spouse, children, others)

Inability to achieve goals in life that one values (marriage, education, children)

Inability to participate in activities one desires (walking, sports)

Loss of something or someone valued (spouse, children, friend, financial resources)

Exposure to long-term physiological or psychological stress

Loss of belief in transcendent values/God

Maturational

Child

Loss of trust in significant other (parents, sibling)

Abandonment by caregivers

Loss of autonomy related to illness (*e.g.,* fracture)

Loss of bodily functions

Inability to achieve developmental tasks (trust, autonomy, initiative, industry)

Adolescent

Loss of significant other (peer, family)

Loss of bodily functions

Change in body image

Inability to achieve developmental task (role identity)

Adult

Impaired bodily functions, loss of body part

Impaired relationships (separation, divorce)

Loss of job, career

Loss of significant others (death of children, spouse)

Inability to achieve developmental tasks (intimacy, commitment, productive)

Elderly

Sensory deficits

Motor deficits

Loss of independence

Loss of significant others, things

Inability to achieve developmental tasks (integrity)

Infection, Potential for

Infection Transmission, Potential for

DEFINITION

Potential for Infection: The state in which an individual is at risk of being invaded by an opportunistic or pathogenic agent (virus, fungus, bacterium, protozoan, or other parasite).

DEFINING CHARACTERISTICS

Major (Must Be Present)

Evidence of risk factors
Altered production of leukocytes
Altered immune response
Altered circulation (lymph, blood)
Presence of favorable conditions for infection (see
Etiological, Contributing, Risk Factors)
History of infection

ETIOLOGICAL, CONTRIBUTING, RISK FACTORS

A variety of health problems and situations can create conditions that would encourage the development of infections. Some common factors are

Pathophysiological

Chronic diseases
Cancer
Renal failure
Arthritis
Hematologic disorders
Diabetes mellitus
Alcoholism
Immunosuppression
Immunodeficiency
Altered or insufficient leukocytes
Blood dyscrasias
Impaired oxygen transport
Altered integumentary system
Periodontal disease
Obesity
Loss of consciousness
Hormonal factors

Hepatic disorders
Respiratory disorders
Collagen diseases
Heritable disorders

Treatment-related

Medications
Antibiotics
Corticosteroids
Antiviral agents
Insulin

Antifungal agents
Tranquilizers
Immunosuppressants

Surgery
Radiation therapy
Dialysis
Total parenteral nutrition

Chemotherapy
Lack of immunizations
Presence of invasive lines
(*e.g.,* IVs, Foley
catheter)

Situational (Personal, Environmental)

Prolonged immobility
Trauma (accidental, intentional)
Postpartum period
Contact with contagious agents (nosocomial or
community acquired)
Postoperative period
Increased hospital length of stay
Malnutrition
Stress
Bites (animal, insect, human)
Thermal injuries
Warm, moist, dark environment (skinfolds, casts)
Inadequate personal hygiene

Maturational

Newborns
Lack of maternal antibodies (dependent on maternal
exposure)
Lack of normal flora
Open wounds (umbilical, circumcision)
Immature immune system
Infants/children
Lack of immunization
Elderly
Debilitated
Immune response decreased
Chronic diseases

Infection Transmission, Potential for

DEFINITION

Potential for Infection Transmission: The state in which an
individual is at risk for transferring a pathogenic agent to
others.

DEFINING CHARACTERISTICS

Major (Must Be Present)

Presence of a pathogen (individual, environmental)

Minor (May Be Present)

Personal habits of the individual

ETIOLOGICAL, CONTRIBUTING, RISK FACTORS

Pathophysiological

Colonization with highly antibiotic-resistant organism

Airborne transmission exposure

Contact transmission exposure (direct, indirect, contact droplet)

Vehicle transmission exposure

Vector-borne transmission exposure

Treatment-related

Contaminated or dirty surgerical procedures (incision and drainage, traumatic wound)

Drainage devices (urinary, chest tubes)

Suction equipment

Invasive devices (endotracheal tubes)

Situational (Personal, Environmental)

Disaster with hazardous infectious material

Unsanitary living conditions (sewage, personal hygiene)

Areas considered high risk for vector-borne diseases (malaria, rabies, bubonic plague)

Areas considered high risk for vehicle-borne disease (hepatitis A, shigella, salmonella)

Maturational

Newborn

Birth outside a hospital setting in an uncontrolled environment

Exposure during prenatal or perinatal period to communicable disease via mother

Injury, Potential for

DEFINITION

Potential for.Injury: The state in which an individual is at risk for injury because of a perceptual or physiological deficit, a lack of awareness of hazards, or maturational age.

DEFINING CHARACTERISTICS

Major (Must Be Present)

Presence of risk factors such as
Evidence of environmental hazards*
Lack of knowledge of environmental hazards
Lack of knowledge of safety precautions
History of accidents
Impaired mobility
Sensory deficits

ETIOLOGICAL, CONTRIBUTING, RISK FACTORS

Pathophysiological

Altered cerebral function
Tissue hypoxia
Post-trauma
Vertigo
Altered mobility
Unsteady gait
Impaired sensory function
Vision
Hearing
Pain
Fatigue
Orthostatic hypotension

Syncope
Confusion

Loss of limb

Thermal/touch
Smell

* See *Etiological, Contributing, Risk Factors* for specific hazards.

Diabetes mellitus
Vertebrobasilar insufficiency
Cervical spondylosis
Subclavian steal
Vestibular disorders
Carotid sinus syncope

Treatment-related

Medications
  Sedatives   Hypogycemics
  Vasodilators   Diuretics
  Antihypertensives   Phenothiazines

Situational (Personal, Environmental)

Decrease in or loss of short-term memory
Dehydration (*e.g.,* summer)
Prolonged bed rest
Stress
Vasovagal reflex
Faulty judgment
Alcohol
Poisons (plants, toxic chemicals)
Household hazards
  Unsafe walkways   Faulty electric wires
  Unsafe toys   Improperly stored
                               poisons
Automotive hazards
  Lack of use of seatbelts   Mechanically unsafe
    or child seats   vehicle
Fire hazards
  Smoking in bed   Improperly stored
  Gas leaks   petroleum
                               products
Unfamiliar setting (hospital, nursing home)
Improper footwear
Inattentive caretaker
Improper use of aids (crutches, canes, walkers,
  wheelchairs)
Environmental hazards (home, school, hospital)

Maturational

Infant/child
  High risk for maturational age
    Suffocation hazards (improper crib, pillow in crib,

plastic bags, unattended in water—bath, pool,
choking on such things as toys or food)
Improper use of bicycles, kitchen utensils/
appliances, sports equipment, lawn equipment
Poison (plants, cleaning agents, medications)
Fire (matches, fireplace, stove)
Falls
Adolescent
Automobile
Bicycle
Alcohol
Drugs
Adult
Automobile
Alcohol
Elderly
Motor and sensory deficits
Medication (accidental overdose, sedation)
Arteriosclerosis

Knowledge Deficit

DEFINITION

Knowledge Deficit: The state in which the individual experiences a deficiency in cognitive knowledge or psychomotor skills necessary for management of a health problem.

DEFINING CHARACTERISTICS

Major (Must Be Present)

Verbalizes a deficiency in knowledge or skill/request for
information
Expresses "inaccurate" perception of health status
Does not correctly perform a desired or prescribed
health behavior

Minor (May Be Present)

Lack of integration of treatment plan into daily
activities

Exhibits or expresses psychological alteration (*e.g.*, anxiety, depression) resulting from misinformation or lack of information

ETIOLOGICAL, CONTRIBUTING, RISK FACTORS

A variety of factors can produce knowledge deficits. Some common causes are listed below.

Pathophysiological

Any existing or new medical condition, regardless of the severity of illness

Treatment-related

Lack of previous exposure
Complex regimen

Situational (Personal, Environmental)

Lack of exposure to the experience
Language differences
Information misinterpretation
Personal characteristics
    Lack of motivation
    Lack of education or
        readiness

Ineffective coping patterns (*e.g.*, anxiety, depression, nonproductive denial of situation, avoidance coping)

Maturational

Lack of education of age-related factors. Examples include

Children
    Sexuality and sexual
        development
    Safety hazards

Substance abuse
Nutrition

Adolescents
    Same as children
    Automobile safety
        practices

Substance abuse (alcohol, other drugs, tobacco)
Health maintenance practices

Adults
  Parenthood
  Sexual function

Safety practices
Health maintenance
  practices

Elderly
  Effects of aging

Sensory deficits

Mobility, Impaired Physical

DEFINITION

Impaired Physical Mobility: A state in which the individual experiences or is at risk of experiencing limitation of physical movement.

DEFINING CHARACTERISTICS

Major (Must Be Present)

Inability to move purposefully within the environment, including bed mobility, transfers, ambulation
or
Inability to move because of imposed restrictions (*e.g.,* bed rest, mechanical and medical protocols)

Minor (May Be Present)

Range-of-motion limitations
Limited muscle strength or control
Impaired coordination

ETIOLOGICAL, CONTRIBUTING, RISK FACTORS

Pathophysiological

Neuromuscular impairment
  Autoimmune alterations (multiple sclerosis, arthritis)
  Nervous system diseases (parkinsonism, myasthenia gravis)

Muscular dystrophy
Partial or total paralysis (spinal cord injury, stroke)
Central nervous system (CNS) tumor
Increased intracranial pressure
Sensory deficits
Musculoskeletal impairment
Spasms
Flaccidity, atrophy, weakness
Connective-tissue disease (systemic lupus
erythematosus)
Edema (increased synovial fluid)

Treatment-related

Bed rest
External devices (casts or splints, braces, IV tubing)
Surgical procedures (amputation)

Situational (Personal, Environmental)

Trauma or surgical procedures
Nonfunctioning or missing limbs (fractures)
Pain

Maturational

Elderly
Decreased motor agility
Muscle weakness

Noncompliance

DEFINITION

Noncompliance: The state in which an individual desires to
comply but factors are present that deter adherence to
health-related advice given by health professionals.

DEFINING CHARACTERISTICS

Major (Must Be Present)

Verbalization of noncompliance or nonparticipation or
confusion about therapy

Direct observation of behavior indicating
noncompliance

Minor (May Be Present)

Missed appointments
Partially used or unused medications
Persistence of symptoms
Progression of disease process
Occurrence of undesired outcomes (postoperative
morbidity, pregnancy, obesity, addiction,
regression during rehabilitation)

ETIOLOGICAL, CONTRIBUTING, RISK FACTORS

Pathophysiological

Impaired ability to perform tasks because of disability
(*e.g.*, poor memory, motor and sensory deficits)
Chronic nature of illness
Increasing amount of disease-related symptoms despite
adherence to advised regimen

Treatment-related

Side-effects of therapy
Previous unsuccessful experiences with advised regimen
Impersonal aspects of referral process
Nontherapeutic environment
Complex, unsupervised, or prolonged therapy
Financial cost of therapy
Nontherapeutic relationship between client and nurse

Situational (Personal, Environmental)

Concurrent illness of family member
Inclement weather keeping client from keeping
appointment
Nonsupportive family, peers, community
Knowledge deficit
Lack of autonomy in health-seeking behavior
Health beliefs run counter to professional advice
Poor self-esteem
Disturbance in body image

Maturational

The developmental maturity of the client is incompatible with the use of the nursing diagnosis *Noncompliance,* which describes the individual who desires to comply, but the presence of certain factors prevents him from doing so. The nurse must attempt to reduce or eliminate these factors for the interventions to be successful. However, the nurse is cautioned against using the diagnosis of *Noncompliance* to describe an individual who has made an informed, autonomous decision not to comply.

Nutrition, Alterations in: Less Than Body Requirements

Impaired Swallowing

DEFINITION

Alteration in Nutrition: Less Than Body Requirements: The state in which an individual who is not NPO experiences or is at risk of experiencing reduced weight related to inadequate intake of nutrients.*

* This diagnostic category describes individuals who can ingest food but only in less-than-adequate amounts. This category should not be used to describe individuals who are NPO or cannot ingest food. These situations should be described by the collaborative problem of

Potential complication:

Electrolyte imbalances

Negative nitrogen balance

Nurses monitor to detect complications of an NPO state and confer with physicians for parenteral therapy. Some nursing diagnoses that may relate to an individual who is NPO are *Potential Alteration in Oral Mucous Membrane* and *Altered Comfort.*

DEFINING CHARACTERISTICS

Major (Must Be Present)

Reported inadequate food intake less than
recommended daily allowance (RDA) with or
without weight loss
Actual or potential metabolic needs in excess of intake

Minor (May Be Present)

Weight 10% to 20% or below ideal for height and frame
Triceps skin fold, mid-arm circumference, and mid-arm
muscle circumference less than 60% standard
measurement
Tachycardia on minimal exercise and bradycardia at
rest
Muscle weakness and tenderness
Mental irritability or confusion
Decreased serum albumin
Decreased serum transferrin or iron-binding capacity
Decreased lymphocyte count

ETIOLOGICAL, CONTRIBUTING, RISK FACTORS

Pathophysiological

Hyperanabolic/Catabolic States
Burns (postacute phase)   Cancer
Infection   Trauma
Chemical dependence
Dysphagia
Cerebrovascular   Parkinson's disease
accident   Neuromuscular
Amyotrophic lateral   disorders
sclerosis   Muscular dystrophy
Cerebral palsy
Absorptive disorders
Crohn's disease   Intestinal obstruction
Cystic fibrosis   (ileus)
Stomatitis
Trauma
Altered level of consciousness

Treatment-related

Medications (cancer chemotherapy)
Surgical reconstruction of the mouth
Wired jaw
Radiation therapy

Situational (Personal, Environmental)

Anorexia
Depression
Stress
Social isolation
Nausea and vomiting
Allergies
Radiation therapy
Parasites
Inability to procure food (physical limitations; financial or transportation problems)
Lack of knowledge of adequate nutrition
Crash or fad diet
Inability to chew (wired jaw, damaged or missing teeth, ill-fitting dentures)
Diarrhea
Lactose intolerance
Ethnic/religious eating patterns

Maturational

Infants/children
 Congenital anomalies
 Growth spurts
 Developmental eating disorders
Adolescents
 Anorexia nervosa (postacute phase)
Elderly
 Altered sense of taste

Impaired Swallowing

DEFINITION

Impaired Swallowing: The state in which an individual has decreased ability to voluntarily pass fluids and/or solid foods from the mouth to the stomach.

DEFINING CHARACTERISTICS

Major (Must Be Present)

Observed evidence of difficulty in swallowing
Stasis of food in oral cavity

Minor (May Be Present)

Coughing
Choking
Apraxia (ideational, constructional, or visual)
Evidence of aspiration

ETIOLOGICAL, CONTRIBUTING, RISK FACTORS

Pathophysiological

Cleft lip/palate
Neuromuscular disorders (*e.g.,* cerebral palsy, muscular
    dystrophy, amyotrophic lateral sclerosis,
    myasthenia gravis, Guillian-Barré, botulism,
    poliomyelitis)
Neoplastic disease (disease affecting brain and/or brain
    stem)
Vascular diseases (*e.g.,* bulbar and pseudobulbar palsy,
    parkinsonism)
Cerebrovascular accident
Right or left hemispheric damage to the brain
Damage to the 5th, 7th, 9th, 10th, or 11th cranial
    nerves
Tracheoesophageal fistula
Tracheoesophageal tumors, edema

Treatment-related

Surgical reconstruction of the mouth and/or throat
Anesthesia
Mechanical obstruction (tracheostomy tube)

Situational (Personal, Environmental)

Altered level of consciousness
Fatigue
Limited awareness
Altered sense of taste
Irritated oropharyngeal cavity

Maturational

Infants/children
Congenital anomalies
Developmental disorders

Nutrition, Alterations in: More Than Body Requirements

DEFINITION

Alterations in Nutrition: More Than Body Requirements:
The state in which the individual experiences or is at risk
of experiencing weight gain related to an intake in excess
of metabolic requirements.*

DEFINING CHARACTERISTICS

Major (Must Be Present)

Overweight (weight 10% over ideal for height and
frame)
or
Obese (weight 20% or more over ideal for height and
frame)
Triceps skin fold greater than 15 mm in men and 25
mm in women

Minor (May Be Present)

Reported undesirable eating patterns
Intake in excess of metabolic requirements
Sedentary activity patterns

* The individual at risk for weight gain can be described by the
label *Alteration in Nutrition: Potential for More Than Body Requirements.*

ETIOLOGICAL, CONTRIBUTING, RISK FACTORS

Pathophysiological

Altered satiety patterns
Decreased sense of taste and smell

Treatment-related

Medications (corticosteroids)
Radiation (decreased sense of taste and smell)

Situational (Personal, Environmental)

Anxiety, depression, stress, loneliness, boredom, guilt
Sedentary life-style
Pregnancy (at risk to gain more than 25–30 pounds)
Lack of basic nutritional knowledge
Ethnic or cultural values and expectations that
emphasize hearty eating and a hefty body weight

Maturational

Adult/elderly
Decreased activity patterns
Decreased metabolic needs

Parenting, Alterations in

Parental Role, Alterations in

DEFINITION

Alterations in Parenting: The state in which one or more individuals experience a real or potential inability to provide a constructive environment that nurtures the growth and development of his/her/their child (children).*

    * A family's ability to function is at a high risk of developing problems when the child or parent has a condition that increases the stress of the family unit.

    Note: The term *parent* refers to any individual(s) defined as the primary caregiver(s) for a child.

DEFINING CHARACTERISTICS

Major (Must Be Present)

Inappropriate parenting behaviors and/or lack of
parental attachment behavior

Minor (May Be Present)

Frequent verbalization of dissatisfaction or
disappointment with infant/child
Verbalization of frustration of role
Verbalization of perceived or actual inadequacy
Diminished or inappropriate visual, tactile, or auditory
stimulation of infant
Evidence of abuse or neglect of child
Growth and development lag in infant/child

ETIOLOGICAL, CONTRIBUTING, RISK FACTORS

Individuals or families who may be at high risk for
developing or experiencing parenting difficulties

Parent(s)

Single	Addicted to drugs
Adolescent	Terminally ill
Abusive	Acutely disabled
Emotionally disturbed	Accident victim
Alcoholic	

Child

Of unwanted pregnancy	Mentally handicapped
Of undesired gender	Hyperactive
With undesired characteristics	Terminally ill
Physically handicapped	Rebellious

Situational (Personal, Environmental)

Separation from nuclear family
Lack of extended family
Lack of knowledge
Economic problems

Inflation	Unemployment

Relationship problems
   Marital discord   Step-parents
   Divorce   Live-in sexual partner
   Separation   Relocation
Change in family unit
   New child   Relative moves in

Other

History of ineffective relationships with own parents
Parental history of abusive relationship with parents
Unrealistic expectations of child by parent
Unrealistic expectations of self by parent
Unrealistic expectations of parent by child
Unmet psychosocial needs of child by parent
Unmet psychosocial needs of parent by child

Parental Role, Alterations in*

DEFINITION

Alterations in Parental Role: The state in which a parent or primary caregiver experiences or perceives a change in role such as role confusion, conflict, or sense of loss due to external factors (*e.g.,* illness, hospitalization, divorce, separation).

* This diagnostic category describes a parent or parents whose previously effective functioning ability is challenged by external factors. In certain situations, such as illness, role confusion and conflict are expected. This category differs from *Alteration in Parenting,* which describes a parent or parents that demonstrate or are at high risk of demonstrating inappropriate parenting behaviors and/or lack of parental attachment. If parents are not assisted in adapting their role to external factors, *Alterations in Parental Role* can lead to *Alteration in Parenting.*

This diagnostic category was developed by the Nursing Diagnosis Discussion Group, Rainbow Babies' and Children's Hospital, University Hospitals of Cleveland.

DEFINING CHARACTERISTICS

Major (Must Be Present)

Parent(s) express concerns about changes in parental role

Demonstrated disruption in care-given routines

Minor (May Be Present)

Parent(s) expresses concerns/feelings of inadequacy to provide for child's physical and emotional needs during hospitalization or in the home.

Parent(s) expresses concern about effect of child's illness on family

Parent(s) expresses concerns about care of siblings at home

Parent(s) expresses guilt about contributing to the child's illness through lack of knowledge, judgment, and so forth

Parent(s) expresses concern about perceived loss of control over decisions relating to the child

Parent(s) reluctant, unable, or unwilling to participate in normal caregiving activities even with encouragement and support

Parent(s) verbalizes/demonstrates feelings of guilt, anger, fear, anxiety, and/or frustration

ETIOLOGICAL, CONTRIBUTING, RISK FACTORS

Situational (Personal, Environmental)

Illness of child

Birth of a child with a congenital defect and/or chronic illness

Hospitalization of a child with an acute or chronic illness

Change in acuity, prognosis, or environment of care (*e.g.,* transfer to or from an ICU)

Invasive or restrictive treatment modalities (*e.g.,* isolation, intubation)

Home care of a child with special needs (*e.g.,* apnea monitoring, postural drainage, hyperalimentation)

Interruptions of family life due to treatment regimen

Separation
  Divorce
  Remarriage
  Death
  Illness of caregiver
Change in family membership
  Birth, adoption
  Addition of relatives (*e.g.*, grandparent, siblings)

Post-trauma Response Syndrome

Rape Trauma Syndrome

DEFINITION

Post-trauma Response: A state in which the individual experiences a sustained painful response to (an) overwhelming traumatic event(s) that has not been assimilated.

DEFINING CHARACTERISTICS

Major (Must Be Present)

Reexperience of the traumatic event, which may be
    identified in cognitive, affective, and/or sensory-
    motor activities
Flashbacks, intrusive thoughts
Repetitive dreams/nightmares
Excessive verbalization of the traumatic events
Survival guilt or guilt about behavior required for
    survival
Painful emotion, self-blame, shame, or sadness
Vulnerability or helplessness, anxiety, or panic
Fear of
    Repetition
    Death
    Loss of bodily control

Anger outburst/rage, startle reaction
Hyperalertness or hypervigilance

Minor (May Be Present)

Psychic/emotional numbness
Impaired interpretation of reality, impaired memory
Confusion, dissociation, or amnesia
Vagueness about traumatic event
Narrowed attention, or inattention/daze
Feeling of numbness, constricted affect
Feeling detached/alienated
Reduced interest in significant activities
Rigid role-adherence or stereo-typed behavior
Altered life-style
Submissiveness, passiveness, or dependency
Self-destructiveness (alcohol/drug abuse, suicide
attempts, reckless driving, illegal activities, etc.)
Difficulty with interpersonal relationships
Development of phobia regarding trauma
Avoidance of situations or activities that arouse
recollection of the trauma
Social isolation/withdrawal, negative self-concept
Sleep disturbances, emotional disturbances
Irritability, poor impulse control, or explosiveness
Loss of faith in people or the world/feeling of
meaninglessness in life
Chronic anxiety or/and chronic depression
Somatic preoccupation/multiple physiological
symptoms

ETIOLOGICAL, CONTRIBUTING, RISK FACTORS

Situational (Personal, Environmental)

Traumatic events of natural origin, including
Floods
Earthquakes
Volcanic eruptions
Storms
Avalanches
Epidemics (may be of human origin)
Other natural disasters, which are overwhelming to
most people

Traumatic events of human origin, such as
  Wars
  Airplane crashes
  Serious car accidents
  Large fires
  Bombing
  Concentration camps
  Torture
  Assault
  Rape
  Industrial disasters (nuclear, chemical, or other life-
    threatening accidents)
  Other traumatic events of human origin that involve
    death and destruction or the threat of them

Rape Trauma Syndrome

DEFINITION

Rape Trauma Syndrome: A state in which the individual
experiences a forced, violent sexual assault (vaginal or anal
penetration) against his or her will and without his or her
consent. The trauma syndrome that develops from this
attack or attempted attack includes an acute phase of
disorganization of the victim and family's life-style and a
long-term process of reorganization of life-style.*

DEFINING CHARACTERISTICS

Major (Must Be Present)
  Reports sexual assault

Minor (May Be Present)
If the victim is a child, parent(s) may experience similar
responses.

Acute Phase
  Somatic responses
    Gastrointestinal irritability (nausea, vomiting,
      anorexia)

* Holmstrom L, Burgess AW: Development of diagnostic categories: Sexual traumas. Am J Nurs 75:1288–1291, 1975

Genitourinary discomfort (pain, pruritus)
Skeletal muscle tension (spasms, pain)
Psychological responses
Denial
Emotional shock
Anger
Fear—of being alone or that the rapist will return (a
child victim will fear punishment, repercussions,
abandonment, rejection)
Guilt
Panic on seeing assailant or scene of attack
Sexual responses
Mistrust of men (if victim is a woman)
Change in sexual behavior

Long-term Phase

Any response of the acute phase may continue if resolution
does not occur.
Psychological responses
Phobias
Nightmares or sleep disturbances
Anxiety
Depression

Powerlessness

DEFINITION

Powerlessness: The state in which an individual perceives
a lack of personal control over certain events or situations.*

* Most individuals are subject to feelings of powerlessness in
varying degrees in various situations. This diagnostic category can
be used to describe individuals who respond to loss of control with
apathy, anger, or depression.

DEFINING CHARACTERISTICS

Major (Must Be Present)

Expresses dissatisfaction over inability to control
situation (*e.g.,* illness, prognosis, care, recovery
rate)

Minor (May Be Present)

Refuses or is reluctant to participate in decision-making

Apathy	Uneasiness
Aggressive behavior	Resignation
Violent behavior	Acting-out behavior
Anxiety	Depression

ETIOLOGICAL, CONTRIBUTING, RISK FACTORS

Pathophysiological

Any disease process—acute or chronic—can contribute to
powerlessness. Some common sources are the following:

Inability to communicate (CVA, Guillain-Barré,
intubation)

Inability to perform activities of daily living (CVA,
cervical trauma, myocardial infarction, pain)

Inability to perform role responsibilities (surgery,
trauma, arthritis)

Progressive debilitating disease (multiple sclerosis,
terminal cancer)

Mental illness

Substance abuse

Obesity

Disfigurement

Situational (Personal, Environmental)

Lack of knowledge

Personal characteristics that highly value control (*e.g.,*
internal locus of control)

Hospital or institutional limitations

Some control relinquished to others	Lack of consultation regarding decisions
No privacy	Social displacement
	Relocation

Altered personal
territory
Social isolation
Lack of explanations
from caregivers

Insufficient finances
Sexual harassment

Maturational

Adolescent
Dependence on peer group
Independence from family
Young adult
Marriage
Pregnancy
Parenthood
Adult
Adolescent children
Physical signs of aging
Career pressures
Divorce
Elderly
Sensory deficits
Motor deficits
Losses (money, significant others)

Respiratory Function, Potential Alteration in

Ineffective Airway Clearance

Ineffective Breathing Patterns

Impaired Gas Exchange

DEFINITION

Potential Alteration in Respiratory Function (AIRF): The
state in which the individual is at risk of experiencing a

threat to the passage of air through the respiratory tract and to the exchange of gases (O_2–CO_2) between the lungs and the vascular system.

Note: This diagnostic category has been added by the author to describe a state in which the entire respiratory system may be affected, not just isolated areas such as airway clearance of gas exchange. Smoking, allergy, and immobility are examples of factors that affect the entire system and thus make it incorrect to say *Impaired Gas Exchange related to immobility,* since immobility also affects airway clearance and breathing patterns. It is advised that *Potential Alteration in Respiratory Function* not be used to describe an actual problem, which is a collaborative problem—not a nursing diagnosis. The three diagnoses—*Ineffective Airway Clearance, Ineffective Breathing Patterns,* and *Impaired Gas Exchange*—can be used when the nurse can definitively alter the contributing factors that are influencing respiratory function; for example, ineffective cough, immobility, or stress. The nurse is cautioned not to use this diagnostic category to describe acute respiratory disorders, which are the primary responsibility of physicians and nurses together (*i.e.,* a collaborative problem). This can be labeled *Potential complication: Acute hypoxia.*

DEFINING CHARACTERISTICS

Major (Must Be Present)

Presence of risk factors that can change respiratory function (see Etiological, Contributing, Risk Factors)

ETIOLOGICAL, CONTRIBUTING, RISK FACTORS

The codes *IGE (Impaired Gas Exchange), IAC (Ineffective Airway Clearance),* and *IBP (Ineffective Breathing Patterns)* are used to indicate factors specific to that diagnosis. Factors without a code relate to all four diagnostic categories.

Pathophysiological

Excessive or thick secretions (IAC)
Infection (IAC, IGE)
Neuromuscular impairment

Diseases of the nervous system (*e.g.,*	Central nervous system (CNS) depression

Guillain-Barré
syndrome,
multiple sclerosis,
myasthenia gravis)
Loss of lung elasticity
COPD (chronic
bronchitis,
emphysema)
Asthma
Decreased lung compliance
Allergic response
Hypertrophy or edema of the upper airway structures—
tonsils, adenoids, sinuses (IAC)

Cerebrovascular
accident (CVA,
stroke)

Aging process

Treatment-related

Medications (narcotics, sedatives, analgesics)
Anesthesia, general or spinal (IAC, IBP)
Suppressed cough reflex (IAC)
Decreased oxygen in the inspired air (IGE)
Bed rest or immobility

Situational (Personal, Environmental)

Surgery or trauma
Pain, fear, anxiety
Fatigue
Mechanical obstruction (IAC)
Improper positioning (IAC)
Altered anatomic structure (IAC)
Tracheostomy
Aspiration
Extreme high or low humidity (IAC, IGE)
Smoking
Mouth breathing (IAC, IBP)
Perception/cognitive impairment (IAC)
Severe nonrelieved cough (IAC, IBP)
Exercise intolerance

Maturational

Neonate
Complicated delivery
Prematurity
Cesarean birth
Low birthweight
Infant/child
Asthma or allergies

Increased emesis (potential for aspiration)
Croup
Cystic fibrosis
Small airway
Elderly
Decreased surfactant in the lungs
Decreased elasticity of the lungs
Immobility
Slowing of reflexes

Ineffective Airway Clearance

DEFINITION

Ineffective Airway Clearance: The state in which the individual experiences a real or potential threat to respiratory status related to inability to cough effectively.

DEFINING CHARACTERISTICS

Major (Must Be Present)

Ineffective cough
Inability to remove airway secretions

Minor (May Be Present)

Abnormal breath sounds
Abnormal respiratory rate, rhythm, depth

ETIOLOGICAL, CONTRIBUTING, RISK FACTORS

See *Potential Alteration in Respiratory Function.*

Ineffective Breathing Patterns*

DEFINITION

Ineffective Breathing Patterns: The state in which the individual experiences an actual or potential loss of adequate ventilation related to an altered breathing pattern.

* This diagnostic category has clinical utility if used to describe situations that nurses definitively treat, such as hyperventilation. Individuals with periodic apnea and hypoventilation have a collaborative problem: *Potential complication: Hypoventilation.*

DEFINING CHARACTERISTICS

(See also *Alterations in Respiratory Function.*)

Major (Must Be Present)

Changes in respiratory rate or pattern (from baseline)
Changes in pulse (rate, rhythm, quality)

Minor (May Be Present)

Orthopnea
Tachypnea, hyperpnea, hyperventilation
Dysrhythmic respirations
Splinted/guarded respirations

ETIOLOGICAL, CONTRIBUTING, RISK FACTORS

See *Potential Alteration in Respiratory Function.*

Impaired Gas Exchange*

DEFINITION

Impaired Gas Exchange: The state in which the individual experiences an actual (or may experience a potential) decreased passage of gases (oxygen and carbon dioxide) between the alveoli of the lungs and the vascular system.

Defining Characteristics

(See also *Potential Alteration in Respiratory Function.*)

Major (Must Be Present)

Dyspnea on exertion

Minor (May Be Present)

Tendency to assume a three-point position (sitting, one hand on each knee, bending forward)

---

* This diagnostic category does not represent a situation for which nurses prescribe definitive treatment. Nurses do not treat impaired gas exchange, but nurses can treat the functional health patterns that decreased oxygenation can affect, such as activity, sleep, nutrition, and sexual function. Refer to *Activity Intolerance.* Nurses also have a responsibility to monitor to detect for physiological complications of hypoxia as a collaborative problem, labeled *Potential complication: Hypoxia.*

Pursed-lip breathing with prolonged expiratory phase
Increased anteroposterior chest diameter, if chronic
Lethargy and fatigue
Increased pulmonary vascular resistance (increased
    pulmonary artery/right ventricular pressure)
Decreased gastric motility, prolonged gastric emptying
Decreased oxygen content, decreased oxygen saturation,
    increased PCO_2, as measured by blood gas studies
Cyanosis

ETIOLOGICAL, CONTRIBUTING, RISK FACTORS

See *Potential Alteration in Respiratory Function.*

Self-care Deficit

DEFINITION

Self-care Deficit: The state in which the individual experiences an impaired motor function or cognitive function, causing a decreased ability to feed, bathe, dress, and/or toilet himself.

DEFINING CHARACTERISTICS

Major (Must Be Present)

1. Self-feeding deficits

Is unable to open food containers
Is unable to cut food
Is unable to bring food to mouth

2. Self-bathing deficits (includes washing entire body, combing hair, brushing teeth, attending to skin and nail care, and applying makeup)

Is unable or unwilling to
    wash body or body
    parts

Is unable to regulate
    temperature or water
    flow

Is unable to obtain water

3. Self-dressing deficits (including donning regular or special clothing—not nightclothes)

Has impaired ability to put on or take off clothing

Is unable to fasten clothing

Is unable to groom self satisfactorily

Is unable to obtain or replace articles of clothing

4. Self-toileting deficits

Is unable or unwilling to get to toilet or commode

Is unable or unwilling to carry out proper hygiene

Is unable to transfer to and from toilet or commode

Is unable to handle clothing to accommodate toileting

Is unable to flush toilet or empty commode

5. Total

Is unable to perform any self-care activities

ETIOLOGICAL, CONTRIBUTING, RISK FACTORS

Pathophysiological

Neuromuscular impairment
  Autoimmune alterations (arthritis, multiple sclerosis)
  Metabolic and endocrine alterations (diabetes mellitus, hypothyroidism)
  Nervous system disorders (parkinsonism, myasthenia gravis, muscular dystrophy, Guillain-Barré syndrome)
  Lack of coordination
  Spasticity or flaccidity
  Muscular weakness
  Partial or total paralysis (spinal cord injury, stroke)
  Central nervous system (CNS) tumors
  Increased intracranial pressure
Musculoskeletal disorders
  Atrophy
  Muscle contractures

Connective tissue diseases
(systemic lupus eryhthematosus)
Edema (increased synovial fluid)
Visual disorders
Glaucoma
Cataracts
Diabetic/hypertensive retinopathy
Ocular histoplasmosis
Cranial nerve neuropathy
Visual field cuts

Treatment-related

External devices (casts, splints, braces, intravenous
equipment)
Surgical procedures

Fractures	Jejunostomy
Tracheostomy	Ileostomy
Gastrostomy	Colostomy

Situational (Personal, Environmental)

Immobility
Trauma
Nonfunctioning or missing limbs
Coma

Maturational

Elderly
Decreased visual and motor ability
Muscle weakness

Self-concept, Disturbance in

DEFINITION

Disturbance in Self-concept: The state in which the individual experiences or is at risk of experiencing a negative state of change about the way he feels, thinks, or views himself. It may include a change in body image, self-esteem, role performance, or personal identity.

DEFINING CHARACTERISTICS

Since a disturbance in self-concept may include a change in any one or combination of its four component parts (body image, self-esteem, role performance, personal identity), and since the nature of the change causing the alteration can be so varied, there is no "typical" response. Reactions may include the following:

Refusal to touch or look at a body part

Refusal to look into a mirror

Unwillingness to discuss a limitation, deformity, or disfigurement.

Refusal to accept rehabilitation efforts

Inappropriate attempts to direct own treatment

Denial of the existence of a deformity or disfigurement

Increasing dependence on others

Signs of grieving
  Weeping
  Despair
  Anger

Refusal to participate in own care or take responsibility for self-care (self-neglect)

Self-destructive behavior (alcohol, drug abuse)

Displaying hostility toward the healthy

Withdrawal from social contacts

Changing usual patterns of responsibility

Showing change in ability to estimate relationship of body to environment

ETIOLOGICAL, CONTRIBUTING, RISK FACTORS

A disturbance in self-concept can occur as a response to a variety of health problems, situations, and conflicts. Some common sources include the following:

Pathophysiological

Loss of body part(s)
Loss of body function(s)
Severe trauma
Chronic disease

Treatment-related

Hospitalization: chronic or terminal illness
Surgery

Situational (Personal, Environmental)
  Divorce, separation from, or death of a significant other
  Loss of job or ability to work
  Pain
  Obesity
  Pregnancy
  Immobility or loss of function
  Need for placement in a nursing home

Maturational
  Infant and preschool
    Deprivation
  Young adult
    Peer pressure
    Puberty
  Middle-aged
    Signs of aging (graying or loss of hair)
    Reduced hormonal levels (menopause)
  Elderly
    Losses (people, function, financial, retirement)

Other
  Women's movement
  Sexual revolution

Self-harm, Potential for*

DEFINITION

Potential for Self-harm: The state in which an individual is at risk for inflicting direct harm on himself.

DEFINING CHARACTERISTICS

Major (Must Be Present)
  Suicidal ideation

  * There is a relationship between *Potential for Self-harm* and *Hopelessness.* Refer to *Hopelessness* for additional information.

Minor (May Be Present)
Severe stress
Depression
Hallucinations/delusions
Hostility
Substance abuse
Low self-esteem
Hopelessness
Acute agitation
Poor impulse control
Lack of a support system
Helplessness

ETIOLOGICAL, CONTRIBUTING, RISK FACTORS

Potential for self-harm can occur as a response to a variety of health problems, situations, and conflicts. Some sources are the following:

Pathophysiological
Terminal illness
Chronic illness (*e.g.,* diabetes, hypertension)
Alcoholism
Organic mental disorder
Ingestion of prescribed or nonprescribed drugs

Treatment-related
Dialysis
Insulin injections or any ongoing treatments
Cancer chemotherapy/radiation

Situational (Personal, Environmental)
Parental/marital conflict
Job loss
Divorce/separation
Threatened or actual financial loss
Alcoholism/drug abuse in family
Wish to reunite with loved one who has died
Depression
Death of significant other
Loss of status, prestige

Someone leaving home
Child abuse
Threat of abandonment by significant other

Maturational

Adolescent
    Separation from family
    Peer pressure
    Role changes
    Identity crisis
    Loss of significant support person
Adult
    Marital conflict
    Parenting
    Loss of family member
    Role changes
Elderly
    Retirement
    Social isolation
    Loss of spouse

Sensory–Perceptual Alteration

DEFINITION

Sensory–Perceptual Alteration: A state in which the individual experiences or is at risk of experiencing a change in the amount, pattern, or interpretation of incoming stimuli.

Note: The category *Sensory–Perceptual Alteration* has six subcategories: visual, auditory, kinesthetic, gustatory, tactile, and olfactory.

When an individual has a visual or hearing deficit, how does the nurse intervene with the diagnosis *Sensory–Perceptual Alteration:*

visual, related to effects of glaucoma? What would the outcome criteria be? The nurse should assess for the individual's response to the visual loss and specifically label the response, not the deficit. Examples of responses to sensory deficits may be the following:

Visual
  Potential for injury
  Self-care deficit
Auditory
  Impaired communicaton
  Social isolation
Kinesthetic
  Potential for injury
Olfactory
  Alteration in nutrition
Tactile
  Potential for injury
Gustatory
  Alteration in nutrition

This diagnostic category differs from the diagnostic category *Alterations in Thought Processes,* which also describes an individual with cognitive alterations, but the stimulus for these alterations comes from within the person's own thoughts, not the external environment.

DEFINING CHARACTERISTICS

Major (Must Be Present)

Inaccurate interpretation of environmental stimuli
Negative change in amount or pattern of incoming
  stimuli

Minor (May Be Present)

Disoriented about time or place
Disoriented about people
Altered problem-solving ability
Altered behavior or communication pattern
Sleep pattern disturbances
Restlessness
Reports auditory or visual hallucinations
Fear
Anxiety
Apathy

ETIOLOGICAL, CONTRIBUTING, RISK FACTORS

Many factors in an individual's life can contribute to sensory–perceptual alterations. Some common factors are listed below.

Pathophysiological

Sensory organ alterations (visual, gustatory, hearing, olfactory, and tactile deficits)

Neurological alterations

Cerebrovascular accident (CVA)	Neuropathies
Encephalitis meningitis	

Metabolic alterations

Fluid and electrolyte imbalance	Acidosis
	Alkalosis
Elevated blood urea nitrogen (BUN)	

Impaired oxygen transport

Cerebral	Respiratory
Cardiac	Anemia

Musculoskeletel changes

Paraplegia	Quadriplegia

Treatment-related

Amputation

Medications (sedatives, tranquilizers)

Surgery (glaucoma, cataract, detached retina)

Physical isolation (reverse isolation, communicable disease, prison)

Radiation therapy

Immobility

Mobility restrictions (bed rest, traction, casts, Stryker frame, Circoelectric bed)

Situational (Personal, Environmental)

Social isolation (patient with terminal or infectious disease)

Pain

Stress

Environment ("noise pollution")

Sexuality Patterns, Altered*

Sexual Dysfunction

DEFINITION

Altered Sexuality Patterns: The state in which an individual experiences or is at risk of experiencing a change in sexual health.†

DEFINING CHARACTERISTICS

Major (Must Be Present)

Identification of sexual difficulties, limitations, or changes

ETIOLOGICAL, CONTRIBUTING, RISK FACTORS

An alteration in sexual patterns can occur as a response to a variety of health problems, situations, and conflicts. Some common sources are indicated below.

Pathophysiological

Endocrine
  Diabetes mellitus
  Decreased hormone
    production
  Myxedema

  Hyperthyroidism
  Addison's disease
  Acromegaly

Note: Altered Sexuality Patterns is a broad diagnostic category that encompasses sexual identity, sexuality, and sexual function. *Sexual Dysfunction* describes dissatisfaction with sexual function.

† According to the World Health Organization, sexual health is "the integration of somatic, emotional, intellectual, and social aspects of sexual being in ways that are enriching and that enhance personality, communication, and love."

Genitourinary
    Chronic renal failure
    Premature or retarded
        ejaculation
    Priapism
    Chronic vaginal
        infection

Decreased vaginal
    lubrication
Vaginismus
Altered structures
Venereal disease

Neuromuscular and skeletal
    Arthritis
    Multiple sclerosis
    Amyotrophic lateral
        sclerosis

Disturbances of the
    nerve supply to the
    brain, spinal cord,
    sensory nerves,
    and autonomic
    nerves

Cardiorespiratory
    Myocardial infarction
    Congestive heart failure

Peripheral vascular
    disorders
Chronic respiratory
    disorders

Cancer
Liver disease

Treatment-related

Medications
Radiation treatment
Altered self-concept from change in appearance
    (trauma, radical surgery)

Situational (Personal, Environmental)

Partner
    Unwilling
    Uninformed
    Abusive
Environment
    Unfamiliar
    No privacy
Stressors
    Job problems
    Financial worries
Lack of knowledge
Fatigue
Obesity
Pain

Not available
Separated
Divorced

Hospital

Conflicting values
Religious conflict

Alcohol ingestion
Drug abuse
Fear of sexual failure
Fear of pregnancy
Depression
Anxiety
Guilt
Fear of sexually transmitted disease

Maturational

Ineffective role models
Negative sexual teaching
Absence of sexual teaching
Aging (separation, isolation)

Sexual Dysfunction

DEFINITION

Sexual Dysfunction: The state in which an individual experiences or is at risk of experiencing a change in sexual function that is viewed as unrewarding or inadequate.

DEFINING CHARACTERISTICS

Major (Must Be Present)

Verbalization of problem with sexual function
Dissatisfaction with sex role (perceived or actual)
or
Reports limitations on sexual performance imposed by
disease or therapy

Minor (May Be Present)

Fears future limitations on sexual performance
Misinformed about sexuality
Lacks knowledge about sexuality and sexual function
Value conflicts involving sexual expression (cultural,
religious)
Altered relationship with significant other

ETIOLOGICAL, CONTRIBUTING, RISK FACTORS

See *Altered Sexuality Patterns.*

Sleep Pattern Disturbance

DEFINITION

Sleep Pattern Disturbance: The state in which the individual experiences or is at risk of experiencing a change in the quantity or quality of his rest pattern as related to his biological and emotional needs.

DEFINING CHARACTERISTICS

Adults

Major (Must Be Present)
Difficulty falling or remaining asleep

Minor (May Be Present)
Fatigue on awakening or during the day
Dozing during the day
Agitation
Mood alterations

Children

Sleep disturbances in children are frequently related to fear, enuresis, or inconsistent responses of parents to the child's requests for changes in sleep rules, such as requests to stay up late.
Reluctance to retire
Frequent awakening during the night
Desire to sleep with parents

ETIOLOGICAL, CONTRIBUTING, RISK FACTORS

Many factors in life can contribute to sleep pattern disturbances. Some common factors are listed below.

Pathophysiological

Impaired oxygen transport
Angina   Respiratory disorders

Peripheral arteriosclerosis — Circulatory disorders

Impaired elimination (bowel or bladder)
Diarrhea — Retention
Constipation — Dysuria
Incontinence — Frequency

Impaired metabolism
Hyperthyroidism — Hepatic disorders
Gastric ulcers

Treatment-related

Immobility (imposed by casts, traction)
Medications
Tranquilizers — Corticosteroids
Sedatives — Soporifics
Hypnotics — Monoamine oxidase
Antidepressants — (MAO) inhibitors
Antihypertensives — Anesthetics
Amphetamines — Barbiturates

Situational (Personal, Environmental)

Lack of exercise
Pain
Anxiety response
Pregnancy
Life-style disruptions
Occupational — Sexual
Emotional — Financial
Social
Environmental changes
Hospitalization (noise, disturbing roommate, fear) — Travel

Social Isolation

DEFINITION

Social Isolation: The state in which the individual experiences a need or desire for contact with others but is unable to make that contact.*

DEFINING CHARACTERISTICS

Since social isolation is a subjective state, all inferences made regarding a person's feelings of aloneness must be validated. Because the causes vary and people show their aloneness in different ways, there are no absolute cues to this diagnosis.

Major (Must Be Present)

Expressed feelings of unexplained dread or
    abandonment
Desire for more social contact

Minor (May Be Present)

Time passing slowly ("Mondays are so long for me")
Inability to concentrate and make decisions
Feelings of uselessness
Doubts about ability to survive
Behavior changes
    Increased irritability or restlessness
    Underactivity (physical or verbal)
    Inability to make decisions
    Increased signs and symptoms of illness (a change
        from previous state of good health)
    Appearing depressed, anxious, or angry
    Postponing important decision-making
    Failure to interact with others nearby
    Sleep disturbance (too much or insomnia)
    Change in eating habits (overeating or anorexia)

ETIOLOGICAL, CONTRIBUTING, RISK FACTORS

A state of social isolation can result from a variety of situations and health problems that are related to a loss of

* Social isolation is a negative state of aloneness. It is a subjective state that exists whenever a person says it does and is perceived as imposed by others. Social isolation is *not* the voluntary solitude that is necessary for personal renewal, nor is it the creative aloneness of the artist or the loneliness—and possible suffering—one may experience as a result of seeking individualism and independence (*e.g.,* moving to a new city, going away to college).

established relationships or to a failure to generate these relationships. Some common sources follow.

Situational (Personal, Environmental)

Death of a significant other

Divorce

Extreme poverty

Hospitalization or terminal illness (dying process)

Moving to another culture (*e.g.*, unfamiliar language)

Drug or alcohol addiction

.Obesity

Cancer (disfiguring surgery of head or neck,
    superstitions of others)

Physical handicaps (paraplegia, amputation, arthritis,
    hemiplegia)

Emotional handicaps (extreme anxiety, depression,
    paranoia, phobias)

Homosexuality

Loss of usual means of transportation

Incontinence (embarrassment, odor)

Communicable diseases (acquired immune deficiency
    syndrome [AIDS], hepatitis)

Maturational

Child

In protective isolation or with a communicable
    disease

Elderly

Sensory losses

Motor losses

Loss of significant others

Social Interactions, Impaired

DEFINITION

Impaired Social Interactions: The state in which individual experiences or is at risk of experiencing negative, insufficient, or unsatisfactory responses from interactions.

DEFINING CHARACTERISTICS

Major (Must Be Present)

Reports inability to establish and/or maintain stable
supportive relationships

Minor (May Be Present)

Lack of motivation
Severe anxiety
Dependent behavior
Hopelessness
Delusions/hallucinations
Disorganized thinking
Lack of self-care skills
Distractibility/inability to concentrate
Social isolation
Superficial relationships
Poor impulse control
Difficulty holding a job
Lack of self-esteem

ETIOLOGICAL, CONTRIBUTING, RISK FACTORS

Impaired social interactions can result from a variety of
situations and health problems that are related to the
inability to establish and maintain rewarding relationships.
Some common sources are as follows:

Pathophysiological

Loss of body function
Hearing deficits
Mental retardation
Terminal illness
Loss of body part
Visual deficits
Speech impediments
Chronic illness (Crohn's disease, renal failure)

Treatment-related

Surgical disfigurement
Dialysis
Medication reaction

Situational (Personal, Environmental)

Depression
Language/cultural barriers
Social isolation
Lack of vocational skills
Substance abuse
Anxiety (phobias)
Divorce/death of spouse
Institutionization
Thought disturbances

Maturational

Child/adolescent
  Altered appearance
  Speech impediments
  Separation from family
Adult
  Loss of ability to practice vocation
Elderly
  Death of spouse
  Retirement

Spiritual Distress

DEFINITION

Spiritual Distress: The state in which the individual experiences or is at risk of experiencing a disturbance in the belief or value system that provides strength, hope, and meaning to his life.

DEFINING CHARACTERISTICS

Major (Must Be Present)

Experiences a disturbance in belief system

Minor (May Be Present)

Questions credibility of belief system
Demonstrates discouragement or despair
Is unable to practice usual religious rituals
Has ambivalent feelings (doubts) about beliefs
Expresses that he has no reason for living
Feels a sense of spiritual emptiness
Shows emotional detachment from self and others
Expresses concern—anger, resentment, fear—over the
    meaning of life, suffering, death
Requests spiritual assistance for a disturbance in belief
    system

ETIOLOGICAL, CONTRIBUTING, RISK FACTORS

Pathophysiological

Loss of body part of function
Terminal illness
Debilitating disease
Pain
Trauma
Miscarriage, stillbirth

Treatment-related

Abortion
Surgery
Blood transfusion
Dietary restrictions
Isolation
Amputation
Medications
Medical procedures

Situational (Personal, Environmental)

Death or illness of significant other
Embarrassment at practicing spiritual rituals
Hospital barriers to practicing spiritual rituals
    Intensive-care
        restrictions
    Confinement to bed or
        room
    Lack of privacy
    Lack of availability of
        special foods/diet
Beliefs opposed by family, peers, health-care providers
Childbirth
Divorce, separation from loved ones

Thought Processes, Alterations in

DEFINITION

Alterations in Thought Processes: A state in which an individual experiences a disruption in such mental activities as conscious thought, reality orientation, problem-solving, judgment, and comprehension related to coping.*

DEFINING CHARACTERISTICS

Major (Must Be Present)

Inaccurate interpretation of stimuli, internal and/or external

Minor (May Be Present)

Cognitive deficits, including abstraction, memory deficits

Suspiciousness

Delusions

Hallucinations

Distractibility

Lack of consensual validation

Language

Confusion/disorientation

ETIOLOGICAL, CONTRIBUTING, RISK FACTORS

Pathophysiological

Personality and mental disorders related to progressive dementia

Alteration in biochemical compounds

Genetic disorder

* This diagnosis differs from the diagnostic category *Sensory-Perceptual Alterations,* which describes an individual with alterations in the amount, pattern, or interpretation of incoming stimuli that are the result of physiological, sensory, motor, or environmental disruptions, whereas, in *Alterations in Thought Processes,* the stimulus comes from within the person's own thoughts, not the external environment.

Situational (Personal, Environmental)

Depression or anxiety
Substance abuse (alcohol, drugs)
Fear of the unknown
Actual loss (of control, routine, income, significant
        others, familiar object or surroundings)
Emotional trauma
Rejection or negative appraisal by others
Negative response from others
Isolation
Unclear communication

Maturational

Adolescent
    Peer pressure
    Conflict
    Separation
Adult
    Marital conflict
    Family additions or deaths
Elderly
    Isolation

Note: These situational and maturational factors should not be considered causative or contributive unless they are present in an individual with a history of coping disorders.

Tissue Integrity, Impaired

Skin Integrity, Impairment of

Oral Mucous Membrane, Alteration in

DEFINITION

Impaired Tissue Integrity: A state in which an individual experiences or is at risk for damage to the integumentary, corneal, or mucous membranous tissues.

Note: *Impaired Tissue Integrity* is the broad category under which the more specific diagnostic categories of *Impairment of Skin Integrity* and *Alterations in Oral Mucous Membranes* fall. Since tissue is composed of epithelium and connective, muscle, and nervous tissue, *Impaired Tissue Integrity* correctly describes some pressure ulcers that are deeper than epithelium. *Impairment of Skin Integrity* should be used to describe potential or actual disruptions of epidermal and dermal tissue only. If an individual is at risk for damage to corneal tissue, the nurse can use the diagnosis *Potential Impaired Tissue Integrity: corneal, related to;* for example: to corneal drying and reduced lacrimal production secondary to unconscious state.

DEFINING CHARACTERISTICS

Major (Must Be Present)

Disruptions of corneal, integumentary, or mucous membranous tissue or invasion of body structure (incision, dermal ulcer, corneal ulcer, oral lesion)

Minor (May Be Present)

Lesions (primary, secondary)
Edema
Erythema
Dry mucous membrane
Leukoplakia
Coated tongue

ETIOLOGICAL, CONTRIBUTING, RISK FACTORS

Pathophysiological

Autoimmune alterations
    Lupus erythematosus   Scleroderma
Metabolic and endocrine alterations
    Diabetes mellitus   Jaundice
    Hepatitis   Cancer
    Cirrhosis   Thyroid dysfunction
    Renal failure
Nutritional alterations
    Obesity   Emaciation

Dehydration   Malnutrition
Edema
Impaired oxygen transport
    Peripheral vascular   Anemia
        alterations   Cardiopulmonary
    Venous stasis   disorders
    Arteriosclerosis
Medications (corticosteroid therapy)
Psoriasis
Eczema
Infections
    Bacterial (impetigo, folliculitis, cellulitis)
    Viral (herpes zoster [shingles], herpes simplex,
        gingivitis, acquired immune deficiency
        syndrome [AIDS])
    Fungal (ringworm [dermatophytosis], athlete's foot,
        vaginitis)
Dental caries/periodontal disease

Treatment-related

NPO status
Therapeutic extremes in body temperature
Therapeutic irradiation
Surgery
Drug therapy (local and systemic)
    Corticosteroids
Imposed immobility related to sedation
Mechanical trauma
    Therapeutic fixation devices
        Wired jaw
        Traction
        Casts
        Orthopedic devices/braces
    Inflatable or foam "donuts"
    Tourniquets
    Footboards
    Restraints
    Dressings, tape, solutions
    External urinary catheters
    Nasogastric tubes
    Endotracheal tubes
    Oral prostheses/braces
    Contact lenses

Situational (Personal, Environmental)

Chemical trauma

Excretions

Secretions

Noxious agents/
substances

Environmental

Radiation—sunburn

Temperature

Humidity

Parasites

Bites (insect, animal)

Inhalants

Poison plants

Immobility

Related to pain; fatigue; motivation; cognitive,
sensory, or motor deficits

Personal

Allergies

Inadequate personal habits (hygiene/dental/dietary/
sleep)

Body build/weight distribution/bony prominences/
muscle mass/range of motion/joint mobility

Stress

Occupation

Pregnancy

Maturational

Infants/children

Diaper rash

Childhood diseases (chickenpox)

Elderly

Dry skin

Thin skin

Loss of skin elasticity

Loss of subcutaneous tissue

Skin Integrity, Impairment of

DEFINITION

Impairment of Skin Integrity: A state in which the individual
experiences or is at risk for damage to the epidermal and
dermal tissue.

DEFINING CHARACTERISTICS

Major (Must Be Present)

Disruptions of epidermal and dermal tissue

Minor (May Be Present)
  Denuded skin
  Erythema
  Lesions (primary, secondary)
  Pruritus

ETIOLOGICAL, CONTRIBUTING, RISK FACTORS

(See *Impaired Tissue Integrity.*)

Oral Mucous Membrane, Alteration in

DEFINITION

Alteration in Oral Mucous Membrane: The state in which an individual experiences or is at risk of experiencing disruptions in the oral cavity.

DEFINING CHARACTERISTICS

Major (Must Be Present)
  Disrupted oral mucous membranes

Minor (May Be Present)

Coated tongue	Leukoplakia
Xerostomia (dry mouth)	Edema
	Hemorrhagic gingivitis
Stomatitis	Purulent drainage
Oral tumors	
Oral lesions	

ETIOLOGICAL, CONTRIBUTING, RISK FACTORS

Pathophysiological
  Diabetes mellitus
  Oral cancer
  Periodontal disease
  Infection
    Herpes simplex   Gingivitis

Treatment-related

NPO 24 hours
Radiation to head or neck
Prolonged use of corticosteroids or other
        immunosuppressives
Use of antineoplastic drugs
Endotrachial intubation
Nasogastric intubation

Situational (Personal, Environmental)

Chemical trauma
  Acidic foods   Alcohol
  Drugs   Tobacco
  Noxious agents
Mechanical trauma
  Broken or jagged teeth   Braces
  Ill-fitting dentures
Malnutrition
  Dehydration
  Mouth breathing
  Inadequate oral hygiene
  Lack of knowledge
  Fractured mandible

Tissue Perfusion, Alteration in

DEFINITION

Alteration in Tissue Perfusion: The state in which the individual experiences or is at risk of experiencing a decrease in nutrition and respiration at the cellular level because of a decrease in capillary blood supply.

Alteration in Tissue Perfusion: Peripheral: The state in which an individual experiences or is at risk of experiencing a decrease in nutrition and respiration at the peripheral cellular level because of a decrease in capillary blood supply.

DEFINING CHARACTERISTICS*

Major (Must Be Present)

Presence of one of the following types:

Claudication   Aching pain

Rest pain

Diminished or absent arterial pulses

Skin color changes

Pallor (arterial)   Reactive hyperemia

Cyanosis (venous)   (arterial)

Skin temperature changes

Cooler (arterial)   Warmer (venous)

Decreased blood pressure changes (arterial)

Capillary refill less than three seconds (arterial)

* Tissue perfusion is dependent upon many physical and physiological factors within the systems of the body and in the structures and functions of the cells. When an alteration in peripheral tissue perfusion exists, the nurse must take into account the nature of the alteration in perfusion. The two major components of the peripheral vascular system are the arterial and the venous systems. Signs, symptoms, etiologies, and nursing interventions are different for problems occurring in each of these two systems and are therefore addressed separately when appropriate.

This diagnostic category is restricted in use to represent only diminished peripheral tissue perfusion situations in which nurses prescribe definitive treatment to reduce, eliminate, or prevent the problem. In the other situations of diminished cardiopulmonary, cerebral, renal, or gastrointestinal tissue perfusion, the nurse should focus on the functional abilities of the individual that are or may be compromised because of the decreased tissue perfusion. The nurse should also monitor to detect for physiological complications of decreased tissue perfusion and label these situations as collaborative problems. The following illustrates examples of a compromised functional health problem (nursing diagnosis) and a potential complication (collaborative problem) for an individual with compromised cerebral tissue perfusion:

Potential for Injury related to vertigo secondary to recent head injury (nursing diagnosis)

Potential complication: Increased Intracranial Pressure (collaborative problem)

Refer to Chapter 2 of Carpenito LJ: Nursing Diagnosis: Application to Clinical Practice, 2nd ed. Philadelphia, JB Lippincott, 1987 for additional information on collaborative problems. For additional examples of nursing diagnoses and collaborative problems grouped under medical conditions, refer to Section II of this handbook.

Minor (May Be Present)

Edema (venous)
Loss of sensory function (arterial)
Loss of motor function (arterial)
Trophic tissue changes (arterial)
    Hard, thick nails
    Loss of hair
    Lack of lanugo (newborn)

ETIOLOGICAL, CONTRIBUTING, RISK FACTORS

Vascular disorders
    Arteriosclerosis
    Hypertension
    Aneurysm
    Arterial thrombosis
    Deep vein thrombosis
    Collagen vascular
        disease
    Rheumatoid arthritis

    Leriche syndrome
    Raynaud's disease/
        syndrome
    Varicosities
    Buerger's disease
    Sickle cell crisis
    Cirrhosis
    Alcoholism

Diabetes Mellitus
Hypotension
    Sympathetic stress response (vasospasm/
        vasoconstriction)
Blood dyscrasias (platelet disorders)
Renal failure
Cancer/tumor
Treatment-related
    Immobilization
    Presence of invasive lines
    Pressure sites/constriction (Ace bandages, stockings)
    Medications (diuretics, tranquilizers, anticoagulants)
    Anesthesia
    Blood vessel trauma or compression
Situational (Personal, Environmental)
    Pregnancy
    Heredity
    Obesity
    Diet (hyperlipidemia)
    Anorexia/Malnutrition
    Dehydration

Dependent venous pooling
Hypothermia
Frequent exposure to vibrating tools/equipment
Tobacco use
Exercise
Maturational
Neonate
Immature peripheral circulation
Rh incompatibility (erythroblastosis fetalis)
Hypothermia
Elderly
Sensory–perceptual changes
Atherosclerotic plaques
Capillary fragility

Unilateral Neglect

DEFINITION

Unilateral Neglect: The state in which an individual is unable to attend to or "ignores" the hemiplegic side of his body and/or objects, persons, or sounds on the affected side of his environment.

DEFINING CHARACTERISTICS

Major (Must Be Present)
Neglect of involved body parts and/or extrapersonal space
Denial of the existence of the affected limb or side of body

Minor (May Be Present)
Left homonymous hemianopsia
Difficulty with spatial–perceptual tasks
Hemiplegia (usually left side)

ETIOLOGICAL, CONTRIBUTING, RISK FACTORS

Pathophysiological

Neurological disease/damage
Cerebrovascular accident (CVA)
Cerebral tumors
Brain injury/trauma
Cerebral aneurysms

Urinary Elimination, Alteration in Patterns of*

Maturational Enuresis

Reflex Incontinence

Stress Incontinence

Total Incontinence

Urge Incontinence

Urinary Retention

* All of these categories pertain to *Alteration in Urinary Elimination,* not urine formulation. Anuria, oliguria, and renal failure should be labeled collaborative problems, such as *Potential complication: Anuria. Alteration in Patterns of Urinary Elimination* represents a broad diagnosis, probably too broad for clinical use. It is recommended that a more specific diagnostic category such as *Stress Incontinence* be used instead. When the etiological or contributing factors have not been identified for incontinence, the diagnosis can temporarily be written *Incontinence related to unknown etiology.*

DEFINITION

Alteration in Patterns of Urinary Elimination: The state in which the individual experiences or is at risk of experiencing urinary dysfunction.

DEFINING CHARACTERISTICS

Major (Must Be Present)

Reports or experiences a urinary elimination problem, such as

Urgency

Frequency

Hesitancy

Nocturia

Enuresis

Dribbling

Bladder distention

Incontinence

Large residual urine volumes

ETIOLOGICAL, CONTRIBUTING, RISK FACTORS

Pathophysiological

Congenital urinary tract anomolies

Strictures

Hypospadias

Epispadias

Ureterocele

Bladder neck contractures

Megalocystis (large-capacity bladder without tone)

Disorders of the urinary tract

Infection

Trauma

Urethritis

Calculi

Carcinoma

Neurogenic disorders or injuries

Cord injury/tumor/infection

Brain injury/tumor/infection

Cerebrovascular accident

Demyelinating diseases

Prostatic enlargement

Multiple sclerosis

Diabetic neuropathy

Alcoholic neuropathy

Tabes dorsalis

Situational (Personal, Environmental)

Post–child birth   Estrogen deficiency
Obesity

Maturational Enuresis

DEFINITION

Maturational Enuresis: The state in which a child experiences involuntary voiding during sleep, which is not pathophysiological in origin.*

DEFINING CHARACTERISTICS

Major (Must Be Present)

Reports or demonstrates episodes of involuntary
voiding during sleep

ETIOLOGICAL, CONTRIBUTING, RISK FACTORS

Situational (Personal, Environmental)

Stressors (school, siblings)
Inattention to bladder cues
Unfamiliar surroundings

Maturational

Child
Small bladder capacity
Lack of motivation
Attention-seeking behavior

Functional Incontinence

DEFINITION

Functional Incontinence: The state in which an individual experiences difficulty in reaching or inability to reach the

---

* This diagnostic category would represent enuresis that is not caused by pathophysiological or structural deficits such as strictures.

toilet prior to urination because of environmental barriers, disorientation, and physical limitations.

DEFINING CHARACTERISTICS

Major (Must Be Present)

Incontinence before or during an attempt to reach the toilet

ETIOLOGICAL, CONTRIBUTING, RISK FACTORS

See *Alteration in Patterns of Urinary Elimination.*

Reflex Incontinence

DEFINITION

Reflex Incontinence: The state in which the individual experiences an involuntary loss of urine caused by damage to the spinal cord between the cortical and sacral (S1–S3) bladder centers.

DEFINING CHARACTERISTICS

Major (Must Be Present)

Uninhibited bladder contractions
Involuntary reflexes produce spontaneous voiding
Partial or complete loss of sensation of bladder fullness or urge to void

ETIOLOGICAL, CONTRIBUTING, RISK FACTORS

See *Alteration in Patterns of Urinary Elimination.*

Stress Incontinence

DEFINITION

Stress Incontinence: The state in which an individual experiences an immediate involuntary loss of urine upon an increase in intra-abdominal pressure.

DEFINING CHARACTERISTICS

Major (Must Be Present)

The individual reports
Loss of urine (usually less than 50 ml) occurring with
increased abdominal pressure from standing,
sneezing, or coughing

ETIOLOGICAL, CONTRIBUTING, RISK FACTORS

See *Alteration in Patterns of Urinary Elimination.*

Total Incontinence

DEFINITION

Total Incontinence: The state in which an individual experiences continuous, unpredictable loss of urine.*

DEFINING CHARACTERISTICS

Major (Must Be Present)

Constant flow of urine without distension
Nocturia more than two times during sleep
Incontinence refractory to other treatments

Minor (May Be Present)

Unaware of bladder cues to void
Unaware of incontinence

ETIOLOGICAL, CONTRIBUTING, RISK FACTORS

See *Alteration in Patterns of Urinary Elimination.*

Urge Incontinence

DEFINITION

Urge Incontinence: The state in which an individual expe-

---

* This category is used only after the other types of incontinence have been ruled out.

riences an involuntary loss of urine associated with a strong sudden desire to void.

DEFINING CHARACTERISTICS

Major (Must Be Present)
Urgency followed by incontinence

ETIOLOGICAL, CONTRIBUTING, RISK FACTORS

See *Alteration in Patterns of Urinary Elimination.*

Urinary Retention

DEFINITION

Urinary Retention: The state in which an individual experiences an inability to void followed by involuntary voiding (overflow incontinence). This category is not recommended for use with individuals with acute episodes of urinary retention (*e.g.,* fecal impaction, postanesthesia, postdelivery), in which cases catheterization, treatment of the cause, or surgery (prostatic hypertrophy) cure urinary retention.

DEFINING CHARACTERISTICS

Major (Must Be Present)
Bladder distention (not related to acute, reversible etiology)
Bladder distention with small frequent voids or dribbling (overflow incontinence)
150 ml or more residual urine

Minor (May Be Present)
The individual states that it feels as though the bladder is not empty after voiding.

ETIOLOGICAL, CONTRIBUTING, RISK FACTORS

See *Alteration in Patterns of Urinary Elimination.*

Violence, Potential for

DEFINITION

Potential for Violence: A state in which an individual is or may be assaultive toward others or the environment.

DEFINING CHARACTERISTICS

Major (Must Be Present)

History of physical harm to others or destruction of property

History of overt aggressive acts

Minor (May Be Present)

Acute agitation

Suspiciousness

Persecutory delusions

Spoken threats of physical assault

Low frustration tolerance

Poor impulse control

Feelings of helplessness

Excessively controlled or inflexible behavior

ETIOLOGICAL, CONTRIBUTING, RISK FACTORS

Pathophysiological

Temporal lobe epilepsy

Progressive central nervous system deterioration (brain tumor)

Head injury

Hormonal imbalance

Viral encephalopathy

Mental retardation

Minimal brain dysfunction

Toxic response to alcohol or drugs

Mania

Treatment-related
Toxic reaction to medication

Situational (Personal, Environmental)
Increase in stressors within a short period
Physical immobility
Suicidal behavior
Environmental controls
Perceived threat to self-esteem
Fear of the unknown
Response to catastrophic event
Rage reaction
Misperceived messages from others
Antisocial character
Response to dysfunctional family throughout
developmental stages
Dysfunctional communication patterns
Drug or alcohol abuse

Maturational
Adolescent
Role identity
Peer pressure
Separation from family

Section II

Medical Diagnostic Categories With Associated Nursing Diagnoses and Collaborative Problems

Medical Diagnoses

Cardiovascular/Hematologic/ Peripheral Vascular Disorders

Cardiac Conditions

ANGINA PECTORIS
Nursing Diagnoses*

Altered Comfort: Chest Pain, related to effects of cardiac ischemia

Fear related to present status and unknown future

Sleep Pattern Disturbances related to treatments and environment

Potential Alterations in Bowel Elimination: Constipation, related to bed rest, change in lifestyle, and medications

Activity Intolerance related to fear of recurrent angina

Potential Disturbances in Self-concept related to perceived or actual role changes

Possible Impaired Home Maintenance Management related to angina or fear of angina

Potential Alteration in Family Processes related to impaired ability of person to assume role responsibilities

Potential Sexual Dysfunction related to fear of angina and altered self-concept

Grieving related to actual or perceived losses secondary to cardiac condition

Knowledge Deficit: (specify)
Examples:

Condition	Diet
Home activities	Medications

* List includes nursing diagnoses that may be associated with the medical diagnosis.

CONGESTIVE HEART FAILURE WITH PULMONARY EDEMA

Collaborative Problems

Potential Complications*
Deep vein thrombosis   *Severe hypoxia*

Nursing Diagnoses

Activity Intolerance related to insufficient oxygen for activities of daily living

Alteration in Nutrition: Less Than Body Requirements, related to nausea; anorexia secondary to venous congestion of gastrointestinal tract and fatigue

Alteration in Tissue Perfusion: Peripheral, related to venous congestion

Anxiety related to breathlessness

Fear related to progressive nature of condition

Potential Impaired Home Maintenance related to inability to perform activities of daily living secondary to breathlessness and fatigue

Self-care Deficit: (specify), related to dyspnea and fatigue

Sleep–Rest Disturbance related to nocturnal dyspnea and inability to assume usual sleep position

Potential Fluid Volume Excess: Edema, related to compensatory kidney mechanisms

Knowledge Deficit: (specify)
  Examples:
    Low-salt diet   Activity program
    Drug therapy (diuretic,   Signs and symptoms of
      digitalis)   complications

ENDOCARDITIS, PERICARDITIS
(Rheumatic, Infectious)

See also Corticosteroid Therapy.
If child, see Rheumatic Fever.

Collaborative Problems

Potential Complications
  Congestive heart failure   *Emboli (pulmonary,*
  Valve stenosis   *cerebral, renal,*
  Cerebrovascular accident   *splenic, heart)*
    (CVA)   *Cardiac tamponade*

---

* Potential complications are collaborative problems, not nursing diagnoses.

Nursing Diagnoses

Activity Intolerance related to insufficient oxygenation
secondary to decreased cardiac output

Potential Alteration in Respiratory Function related to
decreased respiratory depth secondary to pain

Altered Comfort: Pain, related to friction rub and
inflammation process

Knowledge Deficit: (specify)

Examples:

Etiology	Antibiotic prophylaxis
Prevention	Signs and symptoms of complications

MYOCARDIAL INFARCTION (Uncomplicated)

Collaborative Problems

Potential Complications

Dysrhythmias	*Cardiogenic shock*
Cardiac arrest	

Nursing Diagnoses

Altered Comfort: Pain, related to cardiac tissue ischemia

Fear related to present status and unknown future

Sleep Pattern Disturbances related to treatments and
environment

Potential Alterations in Bowel Elimination: Constipation,
related to bed rest, change in life-style, and
medications

Activity Intolerance related to impaired oxygen transport
secondary to decreased cardiac output and fear of
recurrent angina

Potential Disturbances in Self-concept related to perceived
or actual role changes

Possible Impaired Home Maintenance Management
related to angina or fear of angina

Potential Alteration in Family Processes related to
impaired ability of ill person to assume role
responsibilities

Potential Sexual Dysfunction related to fear of angina and
altered self-concept

Grieving related to actual or perceived losses secondary to
cardiac condition

Knowledge Deficit: (specify)
    Examples:
        Condition   Diet
        Home activities   Medications

Hematologic Conditions

ANEMIA

Collaborative Problems

Potential Complications
    Transfusion reaction   *Iron overload (repeated*
    Cardiac failure   *transfusion)*

Nursing Diagnoses

Activity Intolerance related to impaired oxygen transport
    secondary to diminished red blood cell count
Potential for Infection related to decreased resistance
    secondary to tissue hypoxia and/or abnormal white
    blood cells (neutropenia, leukopenia)
Potential for Injury: Bleeding Tendencies, related to
    thrombocytopenia and splenomegaly
Potential Alteration in Oral Mucous Membrane related to
    gastrointestinal mucosal atrophy
Knowledge Deficit: (specify)
    Examples
        Condition   Drug therapy
        Nutritional requirement

APLASTIC ANEMIA

Collaborative Problems

Potential Complications
    Fatal aplasia   *Hypoxia*
    Pancytopenia   *Infection*
    Hemorrhage

Nursing Diagnoses

Activity Intolerance related to insufficient oxygen
    secondary to diminished red blood cell count
Potential for Infection related to increased susceptibility
    secondary to leukopenia

Potential Alteration in Oral Mucous Membrane related to tissue hypoxia and vulnerability

Knowledge Deficit: (specify)

Examples:

Causes	Signs and symptoms of
Prevention	complications

PERNICIOUS ANEMIA

See also Anemia.

Nursing Diagnoses

Alteration in Oral Mucous Membrane related to sore red tongue secondary to papillary atrophy and inflammatory changes

Alteration in Bowel Elimination: Diarrhea/ Constipation, related to gastrointestinal mucosal atrophy

Potential Alteration in Nutrition: Less Than Body Requirements, related to anorexia secondary to sore mouth

Knowledge Deficit: (specify)

Examples

Chronicity of disease	Familial propensity
Vitamin B treatment	

DISSEMINATED INTRAVASCULAR COAGULATION (DIC)

See also Underlying Disorders (e.g., Obstetric, Infections, Burns).
See also Anticoagulant Therapy.

Collaborative Problems

Potential Complications

Hemorrhage	Microthrombi (renal,
Renal failure	cardiac, pulmonary,
	cerebral,
	gastrointestinal)

Nursing Diagnoses

Anxiety/Fear related to treatments, environment, and risk of death

Alteration in Family Processes related to critical nature of the situation and uncertain prognosis

Potential Sensory Perceptual Alterations related to
Examples
Pain
Immobility
Excessive environmental stimuli
Disruption of biorhythms
Knowledge Deficit: (specify)
Examples
Causes   Treatment

POLYCYTHEMIA VERA

Collaborative Problems

Potential Complications
Thrombus formation   *Congestive heart failure*
Hemorrhage   *Peptic ulcer*
Hypertension   *Gout*

Nursing Diagnoses

Alteration in Nutrition: Less Than Body Requirements,
related to anorexia, nausea, and vasocongestion
Activity Intolerance related to insufficient oxygenation
secondary to pulmonary congestion and tissue
hypoxia
Potential for Infection related to hypoxia secondary to
vasocongestion
Knowledge Deficit: (specify)
Examples
Fluid requirements
Exercise program
Signs and symptoms of complications
Thrombi
Congestive heart failure
Hypertension

Peripheral Vascular Conditions

DEEP VEIN THROMBOSIS

See also Anticoagulant Therapy, if indicated.

Collaborative Problem

Potential Complication
  Embolism
  Chronic leg edema
  Chronic stasis ulcers

Nursing Diagnoses

Potential Alteration in Bowel Elimination: Constipation, related to immobility

Potential Alteration in Respiratory Function related to immobility

Potential Alteration in Skin Integrity related to chronic ankle edema

Altered Comfort: Pain, related to impaired circulation (extremities)

Knowledge Deficit: (specify)
  Examples:
    Prevention of recurrence
    Implications of anticoagulant therapy
    Exercise program
    Prevention of sequelae

HYPERTENSION

Collaborative Problems

Potential Complications
  Retinal hemorrhage   *Cerebral hemorrhage*
  Cerebrovascular accident   *Renal failure*
    (CVA)

Nursing Diagnoses

Potential Noncompliance related to negative side-effects of prescribed therapy versus the belief that no treatment is needed without the presence of symptoms

Potential Sexual Dysfunction related to decreased libido or erectile dysfunction secondary to medication side-effects

Knowledge Deficit: (specify)
  Examples
    Diet restriction   Risk factors (obesity,
    Medications   smoking)
    Signs of complications   Follow-up care
                              Stress reduction
                                activities

VARICOSE VEINS

Collaborative Problems

Potential Complications
  Vascular rupture
  Hemorrhage

Nursing Diagnoses

Altered Comfort: Chronic Pain, related to engorgement of
    veins
Knowledge Deficit: (specify)
    Examples:
        Condition
        Treatment options
        Risk factors

PERIPHERAL VASCULAR DISEASE
(Atherosclerosis, Arteriosclerosis)

Collaborative Problems

Potential Complications
  Stroke (CVA)
  Ischemic ulcers
  Claudication
  Acute arterial thrombosis
  Arterial embolization
  Hypertension

Nursing Diagnoses

Alteration in Tissue Perfusion: Peripheral, related to
    compromised circulation
Potential Impaired Tissue Integrity related to
    compromised circulation
Altered Comfort: Pain, related to muscle ischemia during
    prolonged activity
Potential for Injury related to decreased sensation
    secondary to chronic atherosclerosis
Potential for Infection related to compromised circulation
Potential for Injury related to effects of orthostatic
    hypotension
Activity Intolerance related to claudication

Knowledge Deficit: (specify)
> Examples
>> Condition
>> Risk factors
>> Obesity
>> Cold
>> Signs and symptoms of
>>> complications

>> Prevention of
>>> complications
>> Exercise program
>> Foot care
>> Smoking
>> Diet

RAYNAUD'S DISEASE/RAYNAUD'S SYNDROME

Collaborative Problems

Potential Complications
> *Acute arterial occlusion*
> *Ischemic ulcers*
> *Gangrene*

Nursing Diagnoses

Altered Comfort: Acute Pain, related to acute vasospasm
Alteration in Tissue Perfusion related to cold environment
Potential Impaired Tissue Integrity: Ischemic Ulcers,
> related to vasospasm

Fear related to potential loss of work secondary to
> condition

Knowledge Deficit: (specify)
> Examples
>> Condition
>> Stress
>> Cold
>> Stress reduction
>>> techniques

>> Risk factors
>> Smoking
>> Vibrations

STASIS ULCERS (POSTPHLEBITIS SYNDROME)

Collaborative Problems

Potential Complication
> *Cellulitis*

Nursing Diagnoses

Alteration in Tissue Perfusion: Peripheral, related to
> dependent position of legs

Potential for Infection related to compromised circulation
Disturbance in Self-concept related to chronic open
    wounds
Altered Comfort: Chronic Pain, related to ulcers and
    treatments
Knowledge Deficit: (specify)
    Examples
        Etiology of ulcers
        Risk factors
        Prevention of injury, infection
        Exercise program
        Dressings
        Need for compression

Respiratory Disorders

ACUTE RESPIRATORY DISTRESS SYNDROME (ARDS)

See also Mechanical Ventilation (under Diagnostic Studies/ Special Therapies).

Collaborative Problems

Potential Complications
    Electrolyte imbalance   *Hypoxia*
    Of corticosteroid therapy

Nursing Diagnoses

Anxiety related to implications of condition and critical
    care setting
Powerlessness related to condition and treatments
    (ventilator, monitoring)

CHRONIC OBSTRUCTIVE PULMONARY DISEASE—COPD (Emphysema, Bronchitis)

Collaborative Problems

Potential Complications of Hypoxemia/Hypovolemia
    Electrolyte imbalance   *Inadequate cardiac*
    Acid–base imbalance   *output*

Nursing Diagnoses

Ineffective Airway Clearance related to excessive and
    tenacious mucus secretions

Alteration in Nutrition: Less Than Body Requirements,
    related to dyspnea and anorexia

Activity Intolerance related to insufficient oxygenation for
    activities of daily living (ADL)

Impaired Verbal Communication related to dyspnea

Fear related to breathlessness and fear of suffocation

Powerlessness related to loss of control and the
    restrictions that this condition places on life-style

Sleep–Rest Disturbance related to
  Examples
    Cough
    Inability to assume recumbent position
    Environment stimuli

Knowledge Deficit: (specify)
  Examples

Condition	Rest versus activity
Pharmacologic therapy	Breathing exercises
Nutritional therapy	Home care (*e.g.*
Prevention of inflection	equipment)

PLEURAL EFFUSION

*See also Underlying Disorders (congestive heart disease,
cirrhosis, malignancy).*

Collaborative Problems

Potential Complications:

Respiratory failure	*Hypoxia*
Pneumothorax (post-	*Hemothorax*
thoracentesis)	

Nursing Diagnoses

Activity Intolerance related to insufficient oxygenation for
    ADL

Potential Alteration in Nutrition: Less Than Body
    Requirements, related to anorexia secondary to
    pressure on abdominal structures

Altered Comfort: Pain and Dyspnea, related to
    accumulation of fluid in pleural space

Self-care Deficits: (specify), related to fatigue and dyspnea

PNEUMONIA

Collaborative Problems

Potential Complications
Hyperthermia | Septic shock
Respiratory insufficiency | Paralytic ileus

Nursing Diagnoses

Potential Alteration in Body Temperature related to
    infectious process

Activity Intolerance related to insufficient oxygenation for
    ADL

Potential Alteration in Oral Mucous Membrane related to
    mouth breathing and frequent expectorations

Potential Fluid Volume Deficit related to increased
    insensible fluid loss secondary to fever and
    hyperventilation

Potential Alteration in Nutrition: Less Than Body
    Requirements, related to anorexia, dyspnea, and
    abdominal distention secondary to air swallowing

Ineffective Airway Clearance related to pain,
    tracheobronchial secretions, and exudate

Potential for Infection Transmission related to
    communicable nature of the disease

Altered Comfort related to hyperthermia, malaise,
    secondary to pulmonary pathology

Potential Impairment of Skin Integrity related to
    prescribed bed rest

Knowledge Deficit
  Examples
    Fluid requirements | Medication regimen
    Caloric requirements

PULMONARY EMBOLISM

Collaborative Problem

Potential Complication
Anticoagulant therapy

Nursing Diagnoses

Potential Impairment of Skin Integrity related to
    immobility and prescribed bed rest

Knowledge Deficit: (specify)
  Examples
    Anticoagulant therapy   Signs and symptoms of
                                               complications

Metabolic/Endocrine Disorders

ADDISON'S DISEASE

Collaborative Problems

Potential Complications
  Addisonian crisis (shock)   *Hypoglycemia*
  Electrolyte imbalances
      (sodium, potassium)

Nursing Diagnoses

Potential Alteration in Nutrition: Less Than Body
    Requirements, related to anorexia and nausea
Potential Fluid Volume Deficit related to excessive loss of
    sodium and water secondary to polyuria
Alteration in Bowel Elimination: Diarrhea, related to
    increased excretion of sodium and water
Potential Disturbance in Self-concept related to
    appearance changes secondary to increased skin
    pigmentation and decreased axillary and pubic hair
    (female)
Potential for Injury related to postural hypotension
    secondary to fluid/electrolyte imbalances
Knowledge Deficit: (specify)
  Examples
    Disease
    Signs and symptoms of complications
    Risks for crisis
      Infection
      Diarrhea
      Decreased sodium intake
      Diaphoresis
    Overexertion
    Dietary management

Identification (card, medallion)
Emergency kit
Pharmacologic management and titration dose as
needed

ALDOSTERONISM, PRIMARY

Collaborative Problems

Potential Complications
Hypokalemia
Alkalosis

Hypertension
Hypernatremia

Nursing Diagnoses

Alteration in Comfort: Polydipsia, related to excessive
urine excretion
Potential Fluid Volume Deficit related to excessive
urinary excretion
Knowledge Deficit: (specify)
Examples
Condition
Surgical treatment
Corticosteroid therapy

CIRRHOSIS (Laennec's)

See also Substance Abuse, if indicated.

Collaborative Problems

Potential Complications
Hemorrhage
Hypokalemia
Portal systemic
encephalopathy
Negative nitrogen
balance

Drug toxicity (opiates,
short-acting
barbiturates, major
tranquilizers)
Renal failure
Anemia
Esophageal varices

Nursing Diagnoses

Altered Comfort: Pain, related to liver enlargement and
ascites
Alteration in Bowel Elimination: Diarrhea, related to
excessive secretion of fats in stool secondary to liver
dysfunction

Potential for Injury related to decreased prothrombin
production and synthesis of substances used in blood
coagulation

Alteration in Nutrition: Less Than Body Requirements,
related to anorexia, impaired utilization, and storage
of vitamins (A, C, K, D, E)

Potential Alteration in Respiratory Function related to
pressure on diaphragm secondary to ascites

Potential Disturbance in Self-concept related to
appearance changes (jaundice, ascites)

Potential for Infection related to leukopenia secondary to
enlarged, overactive spleen and hypoproteinemia

Altered Comfort: Pruritus, related to accumulation of
bilirubin pigment and bile salts

Fluid Volume Excess: Peripheral Edema, related to portal
hypertension, lowered plasma colloidal osmotic
pressure, and sodium retention

Knowledge Deficit: (specify)
  Examples
    Pharmacologic contraindication
    Nutritional requirements
    Signs and symptoms of complications
    Risks of alcohol ingestion

CUSHING'S SYNDROME

Collaborative Problems

Potential Complications
  Hypertension   *Psychosis*
  Congestive heart failure   *Electrolyte imbalance*
                                  (sodium, potassium)

Nursing Diagnoses

Disturbance in Self-concept related to physicial changes
secondary to disease process (moon face, thinning of
hair, truncal obesity, virilism)

Potential for Infection related to excessive protein
catabolism and depressed leukocytic phagocytosis
secondary to hyperglycemia

Potential for Injury: Fractures, related to osteoporosis

Potential Impairment of Skin Integrity related to loss of
tissue, edema, and dryness

Altered Sexuality Patterns related to loss of libido and
cessation of menses (female) secondary to excessive
adrenocorticotropic hormone production
Knowledge Deficit: (specify)
Examples
Disease
Diet therapy
High protein
Low cholesterol
Low sodium

DIABETES MELLITUS (Adult)

Collaborative Problems

Potential Complications
Hyperglycemia/   Cellulitis
    hypoglycemia   Retinopathy
Neuropathies   Urinary tract infections
Vascular
    (microangiopathy,
    atherosclerosis)

Nursing Diagnoses

Potential Impairment of Skin Integrity related to
increased susceptibility to fungal infection, pruritus
secondary to vascular condition and increased blood
sugar
Potential Sexual Dysfunction (male) related to erectile
problems secondary to peripheral neuropathy
Potential for Injury related to decreased tactile sensation
and diminished visual acuity
Potential for Infection related to depleted host defenses
and depressed leukocytic phagocytosis secondary to
hyperglycemia
Alteration in Nutrition: Greater Than Body
Requirements, related to intake in excess of activity
expenditures
Alteration in Nutrition: Less Than Body Requirements,
related to insufficient coverage for caloric
requirements to maintain growth and development
Potential Noncompliance related to the complexity of
adhering to the prescribed regime

Powerlessness related to the uncertainty of the disease and
the development of complications

Knowledge Deficit: (specify)

Examples

Disease

Nutrition (meal planning)

Weight control

Exercise program

Medications

Type

Administration

Side-effects

Foot care

Signs and symptoms of complications

Record-keeping

Blood/urine testing

Hypoglycemia/hyperglycemia

Detection

Treatment

Community services (support groups)

HEPATITIS (Acute, Viral)

Collaborative Problems

Potential Complications
   Hepatic failure   *Subacute hepatic*
   Coma   *necrosis*
                                    Fulminant hepatitis

Nursing Diagnoses

Activity Intolerance related to fatigue and weakness
secondary to reduced energy metabolism by liver

Potential for Infection Transmission related to contagious
agents

Alteration in Nutrition: Less Than Body Requirements
related to anorexia, epigastric distress, and nausea

Potential Fluid Volume Deficit related to lack of desire to
drink

Altered Comfort: Pruritus, related to bile salt
accumulation

Potential for Injury related to reduced prothrombin
synthesis and reduced vitamin K absorption

Altered Comfort: Pain related to swelling of inflamed liver

Diversional Activity Deficit related to the monotony of
    confinement and isolation precautions
Knowledge Deficit: (specify)
  Examples
    Condition
    Rest requirements
    Precautions to prevent transmission
    Nutritional requirements
    Contraindications
      Certain medications
      Alcohol

HYPERTHYROIDISM

(Thyrotoxicosis, Graves' Disease)

Collaborative Problems

Potential Complications
    Thyroid storm   Cardiac dysrhythmias

Nursing Diagnoses

Alteration in Nutrition: Less Than Body Requirements,
    related to intake less than metabolic needs secondary
    to excessive metabolic rate
Activity Intolerance related to fatigue and exhaustion
    secondary to excessive metabolic rate
Alteration in Bowel Elimination: Diarrhea, related to
    increased peristalsis secondary to excessive metabolic
    rate
Altered Comfort related to heat intolerance and profuse
    diaphoresis
Potential Impaired Tissue Integrity: Corneal, related to
    inability to close eyelids secondary to exophthalmos
Potential for Injury related to tremors
Potential Hyperthemia related to lack of metabolic
    compensatory mechanism secondary to
    hyperthyroidism
Knowledge Deficit: (specify)
  Examples
    Condition
    Treatment regime
    Pharmacologic therapy
    Eye care

Dietary management
Signs and symptoms of complications

HYPOTHYROIDISM (Myxedema)

Collaborative Problems

Potential Complications
Atherosclerotic heart   *Acute organic psychosis*
disease   *Myxedema coma*

Nursing Diagnoses

Alteration in Nutrition: More Than Body Requirements,
    related to intake greater than metabolic needs
    secondary to slowed metabolic rate

Activity Intolerance related to insufficient oxygenation
    secondary to slowed metabolic rate

Alteration in Bowel Elimination: Constipation, related to
    decreased peristaltic action secondary to decreased
    metabolic rate and decreased physical activity

Impairment of Skin Integrity related to edema and
    dryness secondary to decreased metabolic rate and
    infiltration of fluid into interstitial tissues

Altered Comfort related to cold intolerance secondary to
    decreased metabolic rate

Potential Impaired Social Interactions related to
    listlessness and depression

Impaired Verbal Communication related to slowed speech
    secondary to enlarged tongue

Knowledge Deficit: (specify)
    Examples
        Condition   Pharmacologic therapy
        Treatment regimen   Sensitivity to narcotics,
        Dietary management   barbiturates, and
        Signs and symptoms of   anesthetic agents
            complications

OBESITY

Nursing Diagnoses

Alteration in Nutrition: More Than Body
    Requirements, related to intake greater than
    metabolic rate (decreased physical activity)

Ineffective Individual Coping related to increase in food consumption as a response to stressors

Alteration in Health Maintenance related to inadequate exercise program and stress management techniques

Disturbance in Self-concept related to feelings of self-degradation and the response of others to the condition

Knowledge Deficit: (specify)
Examples

Condition	Support groups
Diet therapy	Hazards of overweight condition

PANCREATITIS

Collaborative Problems

Potential Complications

Shock	*Pleural effusion*
Hemorrhagic pancreatitis	*Hypocalcemia*
Respiratory failure	*Hyperglycemia*

Nursing Diagnoses

Altered Comfort: Pain, related to nasogastric suction, distention of pancreatic capsule, and local peritonitis

Potential Fluid Volume Deficit related to decreased intake secondary to nausea and vomiting

Alteration in Nutrition: Less Than Body Requirements, related to vomiting and diet restrictions

Alteration in Bowel Elimination: Diarrhea, related to excessive excretion of fats in stools secondary to insufficient pancreatic enzymes

Knowledge Deficit (specify)
Examples
Disease
Contraindications
Alcohol
Coffee
Large meals
Dietary management
Follow-up care

Gastrointestinal Disorders

ESOPHAGEAL DISORDERS (Esophagitis, Hiatal Hernia)

Collaborative Problems

Potential Complications

    Hemorrhage   *Gastric ulcers*

Nursing Diagnoses

Potential Alteration in Nutrition: Less Than Body
    Requirements, related to anorexia, heartburn, and
    dysphagia

Altered Comfort: Heartburn, related to regurgitation and
    eructation

Knowledge Deficit: (specify)
    Examples

Condition	Positioning after meals
Dietary management	Pharmacologic therapy
Hazards of alcohol and tobacco	Weight reduction (if indicated)

GASTROENTERITIS

Nursing Diagnoses

Potential Fluid Volume Deficit related to vomiting and
    diarrhea

Altered Comfort related to abdominal cramps, diarrhea,
    and vomiting

Knowledge Deficit: (specify)
    Examples

Condition	Signs and symptoms
Dietary restrictions	of complications

HEMORRHOIDS/ANAL FISSURE (Nonsurgical)

Collaborative Problems

Potential Complications

    Bleeding   *Thrombosis*

    Strangulation

Nursing Diagnoses

Altered Comfort related to pain on defecation

Potential Alteration in Bowel Elimination: Constipation, related to fear of pain on defecation

Knowledge Deficit: (specify)

    Examples

        Condition   Exercise program

        Bowel routine   Perianal care

        Diet instructions

INFLAMMATORY INTESTINAL DISORDERS

(Diverticulosis, Diverticulitis, Regional Enteritis, Ulcerative Colitis)

Collaborative Problems

Potential Complications

   Anal fissure   *Anemia*

   Perianal abscess, fissure,   *Intestinal obstruction*

      fistula

Nursing Diagnoses

Altered Comfort: Pain, related to intestinal inflammatory process

Alteration in Bowel Elimination: Diarrhea, related to intestinal inflammatory process

Alteration in Bowel Elimination: Constipation, related to inadequate dietary intake of fiber

Potential Impairment of Skin Integrity (Perineum) related to diarrhea and chemical irritants

Potential Ineffective Individual Coping: Depression, related to the chronicity of the condition and the lack of definitive treatment

Alteration in Nutrition: Less Than Body Requirements, related to diarrhea, dietary restrictions, and pain with or after eating

Alteration in Health Maintenance related to inadequate stress management and exercise program

Knowledge Deficit: (specify)

    Examples

        Condition   Signs and symptoms of

        Dietary restrictions   complications

PEPTIC ULCER

Collaborative Problems

Potential Complications
    Hemorrhage   *Pyloric obstruction*
    Perforation

Nursing Diagnoses

Altered Comfort: Pain, related to lesions secondary to
    increased gastric secretions
Potential Alteration in Bowel Elimination: Constipation,
    related to diet restrictions and side-effects of
    medications
Knowledge Deficit: (specify)
    Examples
        Condition
        Dietary restrictions
        Contraindications
            Certain medications   Tobacco
            Alcohol   Caffeine
        Signs and symptoms of complications

Renal/Urinary Tract Disorders

RENAL FAILURE (Acute)

Collaborative Problems

Potential Complications
    Fluid overload   *Metabolic acidosis*
    Electrolyte imbalance

Nursing Diagnoses

Alteration in Nutrition: Less Than Body Requirements,
    related to anorexia and dietary restrictions
Potential for Infection related to invasive procedures
Knowledge Deficit: (specify)
    Examples
        Disease process   Prognosis
        Treatment   Dietary restrictions

RENAL FAILURE (Chronic, Uremia)

See also Peritoneal Dialysis and Hemodialysis, if indicated.

Collaborative Problems

Potential Complications

Fluid/electrolyte imbalance	*Polyneuropathy (peripheral)*
Hypertension	*Decrease in albumin levels*
Gastrointestinal bleeding	*Congestive heart failure*
Hyperparathyroidism	*Pulmonary edema*
Pathological fractures	*Metabolic acidosis*
Malnutrition	*Pleural effusion*
Anemia, thrombocytopenia	*Pericarditis*

Nursing Diagnoses

Fluid Volume Excess: Peripheral Edema, related to fluid and electrolyte imbalances secondary to renal dysfunction

Alteration in Nutrition: Less Than Body Requirements, related to

Examples

Anorexia	Stomatitis
Nausea/vomiting	Unpalatable diet
Loss of taste, smell	

Sexual Dysfunction related to

Examples

Decreased libido	Amenorrhea
Impotence	Sterility

Disturbance in Self-concept related to effects of limitation on achievement of developmental tasks

Potential Social Isolation (Individual, Family) related to disability and treatment requirements

Altered Comfort related to

Examples

Fatigue	Fluid retention
Headaches	Anemia

Activity Intolerance related to insufficient oxygenation secondary to anemia

Altered Comfort: Pruritus, related to abnormal deposition of calcium secondary to calcium/phosphate imbalance

Powerlessness related to progessively disabling nature of disorder

Knowledge Deficit: (specify)

Examples

Condition

Fluid and sodium restrictions
Dietary restrictions
    Protein
    Potassium
    Sodium
Daily recording
    Intake
    Output
    Weights
Pharmacologic therapy
Signs/symptoms of complications
Follow-up visits
Community resources (support groups)

URINARY TRACT INFECTIONS (Cystitis, Pyelonephritis, Glomerulonephritis)

See also Acute Renal Failure.

Nursing Diagnoses

Altered Comfort: Chronic Pain, related to inflammation
    and tissue trauma
Alteration in Patterns of Urinary Elimination: Dysuria,
    related to inflammation and infection
Potential Alteration in Nutrition: Less Than Body
    Requirements, related to anorexia secondary to
    malaise
Potential Ineffective Individual Coping: Depression,
    related to the chronicity of the condition
Knowledge Deficit: (specify)
    Examples
        Prevention of recurrence
            Adequate fluid intake
            Frequent voiding
            Hygiene measures (personal, post-toileting)
            Voiding after sexual activity
        Signs/symptoms of recurrence
        Pharmacologic therapy

UROLITHIASIS (Renal Calculi)

Collaborative Problems

Potential Complications
    Pyelonephritis   *Acute renal failure*

Nursing Diagnoses

Altered Comfort related to inflammation secondary to irritation of stone

Alteration in Bowel Elimination: Diarrhea, related to renointestinal reflexes

Knowledge Deficit: (specify)
Examples
Prevention of recurrence
Dietary restrictions
Fluid requirements

Neurologic Disorders

BRAIN TUMOR

Because this disorder can cause alterations varying from minimal to profound, the following possible nursing diagnoses reflect individuals with varying degrees of involvement.
See also Surgery (General, Cranial).
See also Cancer.

Collaborative Problems

Potential Complications
Increased intracranial
    pressure
Paralysis
Hyperthermia

Motor losses
Sensory losses
Cognitive losses

Nursing Diagnoses

Potential for Injury related to gait disorders, vertigo and/or visual disturbances, compression/displacement of brain tissue

Anxiety/Fear related to implications of condition and uncertain future

Self-care Deficit: (specify), related to inability to perform/difficulty in performing activities of daily living secondary to sensory-motor impairments

Alteration in Nutrition: Less Than Body Requirements, related to dysphagia and fatigue

Grieving related to actual/perceived loss of function and uncertain future

Impaired Physical Mobility: Upper/Lower Limbs, related to sensory-motor impairment

Altered Comfort: Headache, related to compression/
displacement of brain tissue and increased
intracranial pressure

Alteration in Family Processes related to the nature of the
condition, role disturbances, and uncertain future

Disturbance in Self-concept related to interruption in
achieving/failure to achieve developmental tasks
(childhood, adolescence, young adulthood, middle
age)

Potential Fluid Volume Deficit related to vomiting
secondary to increased intracranial pressure

Potential for Injury related to impaired/uncontrolled
sensory-motor function

CEREBROVASCULAR ACCIDENT

*Because this disorder can cause alterations varying from
minimal to profound, the following possible nursing
diagnoses reflect individuals with varying degrees of
involvement.*

Collaborative Problems

Potential Complications
  Increased intracranial pressure
  Pneumonia
  Atelectasis

Nursing Diagnoses

Sensory–Perceptual Alterations: (specify), related to
hypoxia and compression or displacement of brain
tissue

Impaired Verbal Communication related to dysarthria
and/or aphasia

Potential for Injury related to
  Examples
    Visual field deficits   Inability to perceive
    Motor deficits   Environmental
    Perception deficits   Hazards

Impaired Physical Mobility related to impaired limb
mobility (upper/lower)

Activity Intolerance related to
  Examples
    Fatigue   Inability to tolerate
    Weakness   increased activity

Potential Impairment of Skin Integrity related to
    Examples
        Immobility   Motor deficits
        Incontinence   Nutritional deficits
        Sensory deficits
Incontinence: (specify type), related to
    Examples
        Loss of bladder tone
        Loss of sphincter control
        Inability to perceive bladder cues
Self-care Deficit: (specify), related to (specify)
Impaired Swallowing related to (specify)
Potential Alteration in Bowel Elimination: Constipation,
    related to prolonged periods of immobility,
    inadequate fluid intake, and inadequate nutritional
    intake
Potential Alteration in Respiratory Function related to
    prolonged periods of immobility
Grieving (Family, Individual) related to actual or
    perceived loss of function and inability to meet role
    responsibilities
Potential Impaired Social Interactions related to difficulty
    communicating and embarrassment regarding
    disabilities
Potential Fluid Volume Deficit related to
    Examples
        Dysphagia   Fatigue
        Difficulty in obtaining   Weakness
            fluids   Sensory-motor deficits
Potential Impaired Home Maintenance Management
    related to altered ability to maintain self at home
    secondary to sensory-motor/cognitive deficits
Unilateral Neglect related to (specify site) secondary to
    effects of cerebral pathology
Knowledge Deficit: (specify)
    Examples
        Condition
        Pharmacologic therapy
        Self-care activities of daily living
        Home care
        Speech therapy
        Exercise program
        Community resources
        Self-help groups

Signs and symptoms of complications
Skin care
Bowel/bladder program
Reality orientation
Possible behavioral responses
Lability
Regression

NERVOUS SYSTEM DISORDERS (Degenerative, Demyelinating, Inflammatory; Myasthenia Gravis, Multiple Sclerosis, Muscular Dystrophy, Parkinson's Disease, Guillain-Barré Syndrome, Amyotrophic Lateral Sclerosis)

Because the alterations associated with these disorders can range from minimal to profound, the following possible nursing diagnoses reflect individuals with varying degrees of involvement.

Collaborative Problems

Potential Complications
Renal failure   *Atelectasis*
Pneumonia

Nursing Diagnoses

Disturbance in Self-concept related to prolonged
    debilitating condition and interruption in achieving
    development tasks (adolescence, young adulthood,
    middle age)
Impaired Physical Mobility related to muscle dysfunction
Potential for Injury related to
    Examples
    Visual disturbances   Uncontrolled
    Unsteady gait   movements
    Weakness
Impaired Verbal Communication related to dysarthrias
    secondary to cranial nerve impairment
Potential Alteration in Nutrition: Less Than Body
    Requirements, related to dysphagia/chewing
    difficulties secondary to cranial nerve impairment
Potential Alteration in Bowel Elimination: Constipation,
    related to immobility
Activity Intolerance related to fatigue and difficulty in
    performing activities of daily living

Potential Impairment of Skin Integrity related to
   immobility and sensory-motor deficits
Urinary Retention related to sensory-motor deficits
Grieving (Patient, Family) related to nature of disease and
   uncertain prognosis
Altered Sexuality Pattern (Female) related to loss of
   libido, fatigue, and decreased perineal sensation
Sexual Dysfunction (Male): Impotence, related to
   neurosensory deficits
Potential for Injury related to decreased perception of
   pain, touch, and temperature
Alteration in Family Processes related to nature of
   disease, role disturbances, and uncertain future
Potential Diversional Activity Deficits related to inability
   to perform usual job-related/recreational activities
Potential Social Isolation related to mobility difficulties
   and associated embarrassment
Home Maintenance Management related to inability to
   care for/difficulty in caring for self/home secondary
   to disability or unavailable or inadequate caregiver
Alteration in Parental Role related to disruptions
   secondary to disability
Ineffective Individual Coping: Depression, related to
   implications of disease and its prognosis
Self-care Deficits: (specify), related to
   Examples
      Headaches   Fatigue
      Muscular spasms   Paresis/paralysis
      Joint pain
Powerlessness related to inability to control symptoms
   and the unpredictable nature of the condition (*i.e.,*
   remissions/exacerbations)
Incontinence: (specify type), related to (specify)
Ineffective Airway Clearance related to impaired ability to
   cough
Knowledge Deficit
   Examples
      Condition
      Risks
         Severe fatigue
         Infection
         Cold
         Fever
         Pregnancy

Exercise program
Nutritional requirements
Community services
Medications
  Schedule
  Side-effects

PRESENILE DEMENTIA (Alzheimer's Disease, Huntington's Disease)

See also Nervous System Diseases.*

Nursing Diagnoses

Potential for Injury related to lack of awareness of
  environmental hazard
Alteration in Thought Processes related to an inability
  to evaluate reality secondary to cerebral neuronal
  degeneration
Impaired Physical Mobility related to gait instability
Potential Alteration in Family Processes related to
  effects of condition on relationships, role
  responsibilities, and finances
Impaired Home Maintenance Management related to
  inability to care for/difficulty in caring for self/
  home or inadequate/unavailable caregiver
Unilateral Neglect related to (specify site) secondary to
  neurological pathology
Self-care Deficit: (specify), related to (specify)

SEIZURE DISORDERS (Epilepsy)

*If the client is a child, see also Development Problems/
Needs.*

Nursing Diagnoses

Potential for Injury related to uncontrolled tonic/clonic
  movements during seizure episode
Potential Social Isolation related to fear of a seizure in
  public (embarrassment)

---

* Because these disorders can cause alterations similar to those
in the nervous system disorder category, the reader is referred to
the latter section to review additional possible diagnoses.

Potential Altered Growth and Development related to interruption in achieving/failure to achieve developmental tasks (childhood, adolescence, young adulthood, middle age)

Potential Alteration in Oral Mucous Membrane related to effects of drug therapy on oral tissue

Fear related to unpredictable nature of seizures and embarrassment

Knowledge Deficit:
- Examples
  - Condition
  - Medication
    - Schedule
    - Side-effects
  - Activity versus rest (balance)
  - Care during seizure
  - Community resources
  - Possible environmental hazards
    - Swimming
    - Diving
    - Operating machinery
  - Identification
    - Medallion
    - Card

SPINAL CORD INJURY*

Collaborative Problems

Potential Complications

Accidental extension of injury (acute)
Autonomic dysreflexia (postacute)
Electrolyte imbalance
Spinal shock
Hemorrhage
Respiratory complications
Paralytic ileus

Neurogenic bladder
Hydronephrosis
Gastrointestinal bleeding
Infection (pulmonary, renal)
Thrombophlebitis (deep vein)
Postural hypotension

* Because disabilities associated with spinal cord injuries can be varied (hemiparesis, quadriparesis, diplegia, monoplegia, triplegia, paraplegia), the nurse will have to specify clearly the individual's limitations in the diagnostic statement.

Nursing Diagnoses

Self-care Deficit: (specify), related to sensory-motor
    deficits secondary to level of spinal cord injury

Impaired Verbal Communication related to impaired
    ability to speak words secondary to tracheostomy

Fear related to
  Examples
    Abandonment by others
    Changes in role responsibilities
    Effects of injury on life-style
    Multiple tests and procedures
    Separation from support systems

Grieving: Denial, Anger, Depression, related to
    anticipated losses secondary to sensory-motor deficits

Alteration in Family Processes related to adjustment
    requirements for the situation (time, energy,
    financial, physical care, prognosis)

Potential Impaired Home Maintenance Management
    related to inadequate resources, housing, or impaired
    caregiver(s)

Potential Social Isolation (Individual/Family) related to
    disability or requirements for the caregiver(s)

Potential Alteration in Parenting: Abuse, Rejection,
    Overprotection, related to inadequate resources and
    coping mechanisms

Disturbance in Self-concept related to effects of
    limitations on achievement of developmental tasks

Potential Fluid Volume Deficit related to difficulty
    obtaining liquids

Potential Alterations in Nutrition: More Than Body
    Requirements, related to imbalance of intake versus
    activity expenditures

Potential Alterations in Nutrition: Less Than Body
    Requirements, related to anorexia and increased
    metabolic requirements

Potential Diversional Activity Deficit related to effects of
    limitations on ability to participate in recreational
    activities

Potential Alteration in Bowel Elimination: Constipation,
    related to bowel atony, decreased peristalsis, and
    decreased ability to defecate voluntarily secondary to
    sensory-motor deficits and immobility

Reflex Incontinence or Urinary Retention related to
    bladder atony secondary to sensory-motor deficits

Potential Impairment of Skin Integrity related to
  Examples
    Decreased vascular tone   Sensory-motor deficits
    Immobility   Incontinence (bowel,
                                       bladder)
Potential for Injury related to impaired ability to control
  movements and sensory-motor deficits
Potential for Injury: Fractures, related to bone
  demineralization secondary to immobility
Potential for Infection related to
  Examples
    Urinary stasis
    Repeated catheterizations
    Invasive procedures
      Skeletal tongs
      Tracheostomy
      Venous lines
      Surgical sites
Potential Alteration in Respiratory Function related to
  Examples
    Immobility   Mechanical obstruction
    Excessive secretions
Potential Sexual Dysfunction related to
  Examples
    Inability to achieve or sustain an erection for
      intercourse
    Limitations on sexual performance
    Value conflicts regarding sexual expression
    Depression/anxiety
    Decreased libido
    Altered self-concept
    Unwilling/uninformed partner
Knowledge Deficit: (specify)
  Examples
    Condition   Rehabilitation
    Treatment regimen   Assistance devices

UNCONSCIOUS INDIVIDUAL

See also Mechanical Ventilation, if indicated.

Collaborative Problems

Potential Complications
  Respiratory insufficiency   *Bladder distention*
  Pneumonia   *Seizures*

Atelectasis
Fluid/electrolyte
imbalance
Negative nitrogen
balance

Stress ulcers
Increased intracranial
pressure

Nursing Diagnoses

Potential for Infection related to immobility and invasive devices (tracheostomy, Foley catheter, venous lines)

Potential Impairment of Skin Integrity related to immobility

Potential Impaired Tissue Integrity: Corneal, related to corneal drying secondary to open eyes and lower tear production

Anxiety/Fear (Family) related to present state of individual and uncertain prognosis

Potential Alteration in Oral Mucous Membrane related to inability to perform mouth care on self and pooling of secretions

Self-care Deficit: Total, related to unconscious state

Total Incontinence related to unconscious state

Sensory Disorders

OPHTHALMIC DISORDERS (Cataracts, Detached Retina, Glaucoma, Inflammations)

See also Ophthalmic Surgery, if indicated.

Nursing Diagnoses

Potential for Injury related to impaired vision secondary to condition or eye patches

Altered Comfort: Pain, related to
Examples
Inflammation
Lid
Lacrimal structures
Conjunctiva
Uveal tract
Retina
Cornea
Sclera
Infection

Increased intraocular pressure
Ocular tumors
Potential Social Isolation related to fear of injury or
embarrassment outside home environment
Potential Impaired Home Maintenance Management
related to impaired ability to perform activities of
daily living secondary to impaired vision
Self-care Deficit: (specify), related to impaired vision
Anxiety/Fear related to the actual or possible loss of
vision
Knowledge Deficit: (specify)
Examples
Condition
Eye care
Patches
Compresses
Medications
Eye drops
Instillation
Safety measures
Activity restrictions
Follow-up care

OTIC DISORDERS (Infections, Mastoiditis, Trauma)
Nursing Diagnoses

Potential for Injury related to disturbances of balance
and impaired ability to detect environmental
hazards
Impaired Verbal Communication related to difficulty
understanding others secondary to impaired
hearing
Potential Impaired Social Interactions related to
difficulty in participating in conversations
Social Isolation related to the lack of contact with
others secondary to fear and embarrassment of
hearing losses
Alteration in Comfort: Pain, related to
Examples
Inflammation   Tinnitus
Infection   Vertigo
Anxiety/Fear related to actual or possible loss of
hearing

Knowledge Deficit: (specify)
    Examples
      Condition
      Medications
      Prevention of recurrence
      Hazards
        Swimming
        Air travel
        Showers
      Signs and symptoms of complications
      Hearing aids

Integumentary Disorders

DERMATOLOGIC DISORDERS (Dermatitis, Psoriasis, Eczema)

Nursing Diagnoses

Impairment of Skin Integrity related to lesions and
    inflammatory response
Altered Comfort: Pruritus, related to dermal eruptions
Potential Impaired Social Interaction related to fear of
    embarrassment and negative reactions of others
Potential Disturbance in Self-concept related to
    appearance and response of others
Knowledge Deficit: (specify)
    Examples
      Condition   Contraindications
      Topical agents

PRESSURE ULCERS*

Nursing Diagnoses

Potential for Infection related to susceptibility of open
    wound
Impaired Tissue Integrity: Pressure Ulcers related to
    Examples
      Skin deficits (edema, obesity, dryness)

* The factors that can contribute to the development of pressure
sores are varied and complex; therefore, the nurse must assess for
and identify the specific etiologic/contributing risk factors for the
individual.

Impaired oxygen transport (edema, peripheral anemia)

Chemical/mechanical irritants (casts, radiation, incontinence)

Nutritional deficits

Systemic deficits (infection, cancer, renal or hepatic disorders, diabetes mellitus)

Sensory deficits (confusion, cord injury, neuropathy)

Immobility

Impaired Home Maintenance Management related to complexity of care or unavailable caregiver

The following are some situations that contribute to pressure sore development. If the situation is present in the client, the nursing diagnosis can be used.

Alteration in Nutrition: Less Than Body Requirements, related to anorexia secondary to (specify)

Impaired Physical Mobility related to (specify)

Fluid Volume Excess: Edema, related to (specify)

Total Incontinence related to (specify)

Sensory–Perceptual Alterations: Inability to Feel or Perceive Pressure, related to (specify)

Knowledge Deficit: (specify)

Examples

| Causes of pressure ulcers | Preventive measures Treatment |

SKIN INFECTIONS (Impetigo, Herpes Zoster, Fungal Infections)

Collaborative Problems

Potential Complications (Herpes Zoster)

Post-herpetic neuralgia	Corneal ulceration
Keratitis	Blindness
Uveitis	

Nursing Diagnoses

Impairment of Skin Integrity related to lesions and pruritus

Altered Comfort: Pain, Pruritus, related to dermal eruptions

Potential for Infection Transmission related to contagious nature of the organism

Knowledge Deficit: (specify)
  Examples
    Condition (causes, course)
    Prevention
    Treatments
    Skin care

THERMAL INJURIES (Burns, Severe Hypothermia)

Acute Period
Collaborative Problems

Potential Complications
  Death
  Fluid-loss shock
  Fluid overload
  Infection/septicemia
  Emboli
  Graft rejection
  Hypothermia
  Hypokalemia/
    hyperkalemia
  Curling's ulcer
  Paralytic ileus

  Anemia
  Negative nitrogen
    balance
  Convulsive disorders
  Stress diabetes
  Adrenocortical
    insufficiency
  Pneumonia
  Renal failure
  Compartmental syndrome

Nursing Diagnoses

Impairment of Skin Integrity related to loss of protective
  layer secondary to thermal injury

Alteration in Nutrition: Less Than Body Requirements,
  related to increased caloric requirement secondary to
  thermal injury and inability to ingest increased
  requirements

Altered Comfort: Pain, related to thermal injury and
  treatments

Self-care Deficit: (specify), related to impaired range of
  motion ability secondary to pain and contractures

Fear related to painful procedures and possibility of death

Potential Social Isolation related to infection control
  measures and separation from family and support
  systems

Potential Alteration in Bowel Elimination: Constipation,
  related to immobility and effects of pain medication
  on peristalsis

Sleep Pattern Disturbances related to position restrictions, pain, and treatment interruptions

Potential Sensory–Perceptual Alterations related to
Examples

Excessive environmental stimuli	Imposed immobility
	Sleep deprivation
	Protective isolation
Stress	

Grieving (Family, Individual) related to actual or perceived impact of injury on life (appearance, relationships, occupation)

Potential Impaired Tissue Integrity: Pressure Ulcer, related to immobility

Postacute Period

If individual is a child, see also Developmental Problems/ Needs.

Collaborative Problems

Potential Complications
  Same as in acute period

Nursing Diagnoses

Diversional Activity Deficit related to monotony of confinement

Potential Social Isolation related to embarrassment and the response of others to injury

Powerlessness related to inability to control present situation

Disturbances in Self-concept related to effects of thermal injury on achieving developmental tasks (child, adolescent, adult)

Potential Impaired Physical Mobility: Contractures, related to loss of motion, scarring or reluctance to move secondary to pain

Fear related to uncertain future and effects of injury on life-style, relationships, occupation

Impaired Home Maintenance Management related to long-term requirements of treatments

Knowledge Deficit: (specify)
  Examples
    Condition
    Treatment
      Surgery
      Whirlpool

Nutritional requirements
Pain management
Home care
Rehabilitation
Community services

Musculoskeletal/Connective-Tissue Disorders

FRACTURED JAW

Nursing Diagnoses

Potential Ineffective Airway Clearance related to inadequate cough

Alteration in Oral Mucous Membrane related to difficulty in performing oral hygiene secondary to fixation devices

Impaired Verbal Communication related to fixation devices

Altered Comfort: Pain, related to tissue trauma

Potential Alteration in Nutrition: Less Than Body Requirements, related to inability to ingest solid food secondary to fixation devices

Knowledge Deficit: (specify)
  Examples
    Mouth care
    Nutritional requirements
    Signs and symptoms of infection
    Procedure for emergency wire cutting (*e.g.*, vomiting)

FRACTURES

See also Casts.

Collaborative Problems

Potential Complications
  Neurovascular (paresis, paralysis)
  Fat embolism syndrome
  Shock (hemorrhagic, hypovolemic)
  Misalignment
  Osteomyelitis
  Compartmental syndrome
  Contracture

Nursing Diagnoses

Altered Comfort: Pain, related to tissue trauma

Potential Impairment of Skin Integrity related to
mechanical irritants/compression secondary to casts
and traction

Potential for Infection related to invasive fixation devices

Self-care Deficits: (specify), related to impaired ability to
use upper/lower limb secondary to immobilization
device

Diversional Activity Deficit related to boredom of
confinement secondary to immobilization devices

Potential for Infection: Urinary Tract, related to
immobility secondary to fixation devices

Potential Impaired Home Maintenance Management
related to

   Examples

Fixation device	Unavailable support
Impaired physical	system
mobility	

Alteration in Family Processes related to difficulty of ill
person in assuming role responsibilities secondary to
limited motion

Potential Alteration in Bowel Elimination: Constipation,
related to decreased physical activity

Potential Alteration in Respiratory Function related to
immobility secondary to traction or other fixation
devices

Knowledge Deficit: (specify)

   Examples

     Condition

     Cast care

     Use of assistive devices

       Cane

       Crutches

       Walker

     Signs and symptoms of complications

       Numbness

       Pallor

       Decreased sensation

     Limitations

LOW BACK PAIN

Collaborative Problems

Potential Complications
  Herniated nucleus pulposus

Nursing Diagnoses

Altered Comfort: Pain, related to
  Examples

Acute lumbosacral strain	Osteoarthritis of spine
	Spinal stenosis
Unstable lumbosacral ligaments	Intervertebral disk problem
Weak muscles	

Impaired Physical Mobility related to decreased mobility
  and flexibility secondary to muscle spasm
Potential Ineffective Individual Coping: Depression,
  related to effects of chronic pain on life-style
Potential Alteration in Family Processes related to
  impaired ability of individual to meet role
  responsibilities (financial, home, social)
Knowledge Deficit: (specify)
  Examples
    Condition
    Exercise program
    Noninvasive pain relief methods
      Relaxation
      Imagery
    Proper posture and body mechanics

OSTEOMYELITIS

Collaborative Problems

Potential Complications
  Bone abscess

Nursing Diagnoses

Altered Comfort: Pain, related to soft tissue edema
  secondary to infection
Impaired Physical Mobility related to limited range of
  motion of affected bone
Knowledge Deficit: (specify)
  Examples
    Condition
      Etiology
      Course
    Pharmacologic therapy
    Nutritional requirements
    Pain management
    Signs and symptoms of complications

OSTEOPOROSIS

Collaborative Problems

Potential Complications
    Fractures   *Paralytic ileus*
    Kyphosis

Nursing Diagnoses

Altered Comfort: Pain, related to muscle spasm and
    fractures

Alteration in Health Maintenance related to insufficient
    daily physical activity

Alteration in Nutrition: Less Than Body Requirements,
    related to inadequate dietary intake of calcium,
    protein, and vitamin D

Impaired Physical Mobility related to limited range of
    motion secondary to skeletal changes

Fear related to unpredictable nature of condition

Potential for Injury: Fractures, related to porous bones
    secondary to disease process

Knowledge Deficit: (specify)
    Examples
        Condition
            Etiology
            Course
        Nutritional therapy
        Activity program
        Safety precautions
        Prevention

RHEUMATIC DISEASES

Nursing Diagnoses

Altered Comfort: Pain, related to inflammatory
    response and joint immobility (stiffness)

Activity Intolerance related to fatigue and stiffness

Self-care Deficits: (specify), related to loss of motion,
    muscle weakness, pain, stiffness, or fatigue

Ineffective Individual Coping related to the stress
    imposed by exacerbations (unpredictable)

Health Maintenance: Stress Management

Disturbances in Self-concept related to physical and
    psychological changes imposed by the disease

Impaired Home Maintenance Management related to
impaired ability to perform household
responsibilities secondary to limited mobility

Sleep Pattern Disturbance related to pain

Impaired Home Maintenance Management related to
fatigue and impaired mobility

Impaired Physical Mobility related to pain and limited
motion of limbs

Sexual Dysfunction related to difficulty assuming
position (female), fatigue, or pain

Potential Social Isolation related to ambulation
difficulty and fatigue

Alteration in Family Processes related to difficulty in
assuming/inability to assume role responsibilities
secondary to fatigue and limited motion

Knowledge Deficit: (specify)

Examples

Condition	Quackery
Rest vs. exercise	Heat therapy
Self-help groups	Pharmacologic
Assistive devices	therapy

Infectious/Immunodeficient Disorders

LUPUS ERYTHEMATOSUS (Systemic)

See also Rheumatic Diseases.
See also Corticosteroid Therapy.

Collaborative Problems

Potential Complications
Renal failure secondary to corticosteroid therapy
Pericarditis
Pleuritis

Nursing Diagnoses

Powerlessness related to unpredictable course (remissions,
exacerbations)

Ineffective Individual Coping: Depression, related to
unpredictable course and altered appearance

Potential Social Isolation related to embarrassment and
the response of others to appearance

Potential Disturbance in Self-concept related to inability to achieve developmental tasks secondary to disabling condition

Knowledge Deficit: (specify)
Examples
Condition   Pharmacologic therapy
Rest/activity balance

MENINGITIS/ENCEPHALITIS

Collaborative Problems

Potential Complications
Fluid/electrolyte   Seizures
    imbalance   Septicemia
Cerebral edema   Alkalosis
Adrenal damage   Increased intracranial
Circulatory collapse   pressure
Hemorrhage

Nursing Diagnoses

Potential for Infection transmission related to contagious nature of organism

Altered Comfort: Headache, Fever, Neck Pain, related to meningeal irritation

Activity Intolerance related to fatigue and malaise secondary to infection

Potential Impairment of Skin Integrity related to immobility, dehydration, and diaphoresis

Potential Alteration in Oral Mucous Membrane related to dehydration and impaired ability to perform mouth care

Potential Alteration in Nutrition: Less Than Body Requirements, related to anorexia, fatigue, nausea, and vomiting

Potential Alteration in Respiratory Function related to immobility and pain

Potential for Injury related to restlessness and disorientation secondary to meningeal irritation

Alteration in Family Processes related to critical nature of situation and uncertain prognosis

Anxiety/Fear related to treatments, environment, and risk of death

Knowledge Deficit: (specify)
   Examples
      Condition
      Treatments
      Pharmacologic therapy
      Rest/activity balance

      Signs and symptoms of
        complications
      Follow-up care
      Prevention of
        recurrence

SEXUALLY TRANSMITTED INFECTIOUS DISEASES (Venereal Diseases, Herpes, Acquired Immune Deficiency Syndrome [AIDS])

Nursing Diagnoses

Potential for Infection Transmission related to
    contagious agents
Fear related to nature of the condition and its
    implications for life-style
Grieving related to chronicity of condition (herpes) or
    poor prognosis (AIDS)
Altered Comfort related to inflammatory process
Hopelessness related to incurable nature of condition
Social Isolation related to fear of transmitting disease to
    others
Knowledge Deficit: (specify)
   Examples
      Condition
      Modes of transmission
      Consequences of repeated infections
      Prevention of recurrences

Neoplastic Disorders

CANCER (General)

Nursing Diagnoses

Alteration in Oral Mucous Membranes related to
   Examples
      Disease process
      Therapy
        Radiation
        Chemotherapy

Inadequate oral hygiene
Altered nutritional/hydration status
Potential Sexual Dysfunction related to (specify) or
Potential Altered Sexuality Patterns
Examples
Fear
Grieving
Changes in body image
Anatomical changes
Pain, fatigue (treatments, disease)
Change in role responsibilities
Altered Comfort related to disease process and
treatments
Alteration in Bowel Elimination: Diarrhea, related to
Examples

Disease process	Radiation
Chemotherapy	Medications

Alteration in Bowel Elimination: Constipation, related
to
Examples

Disease process	Immobility
Chemotherapy	Dietary intake
Radiation therapy	Medications

Disturbance in Self-concept related to
Examples

Anatomical changes	Uncertain future
Role disturbances	Disruption of life-style

Self-care Deficits: (specify), related to fatigue, pain, or
depression
Potential for Infection related to altered immune
system
Alteration in Nutrition: Less Than Body Requirements,
related to anorexia, fatigue, nausea, and vomiting
secondary to disease process and treatments
Potential for Injury: Physical Falls, related to
Examples
Disorientation
Weakness
Sensory/perceptual deterioration
Skeletal/muscle deterioration
Potential Impairment of Skin Integrity related to
Examples

Immobility	Altered sensation

Altered nutrition
  status
Altered circulation
Excretions/secretions
Radiation therapy

Potential Fluid Volume Deficit related to
  Examples
    Altered ability/desire
      to obtain fluids
    Weakness
    Vomiting
    Diarrhea
    Depression
    Fatigue

Potential Impaired Home Maintenance Management
    related to
  Examples
    Lack of knowledge
    Lack of resources
      Support system
      Equipment
      Finances
    Motor deficits
    Sensory deficits
    Cognitive deficits
    Emotional deficits

Potential Impaired Social Interactions related to fear of
    rejection or actual rejection of others after
    diagnosis

Potential for Injury related to bleeding tendencies and
    thrombocytopenia

Potential Alteration in Respiratory Function related to
    fatigue, pain, and immobility

Powerlessness related to inability to control situation

Alteration in Family Process related to
  Examples
    Stress of diagnosis/
      treatments
    Role disturbances
    Uncertain future

Grieving (Family, Individual) related to actual,
    perceived, or anticipated losses associated with
    diagnosis

Knowledge Deficit: (specify)
  Examples

    Disease
    Misconceptions
    Treatments
    Home care
    Support agencies
      Self-help groups

American Cancer Society
Hospital associations

COLORECTAL CANCER
(Additional Nursing Diagnoses)

See also Cancer (General).

Potential Sexual Dysfunction (Male) related to inability
to have or sustain an erection secondary to
surgical procedure on perineal structures

Knowledge Deficit: (specify)
Examples
Preoperative procedures
Postoperative procedures
Ostomy care
Appliances
Irrigations
Dietary management
Signs and symptoms of complications

Surgical Procedures

GENERAL SURGERY

Preoperative Period
Nursing Diagnoses

Anxiety related to surgical experience and the
unpredictable outcome

Knowledge Deficit: (specify)
Examples
Preoperative procedures
Surgical permit
Diagnostic studies
Foley catheter
Diet and fluid restrictions
Medications

    Skin preparation
    Waiting area for family
  Postoperative procedure
    Disposition (recovery room, intensive care unit)
    Medications for pain
    Coughing-turning-leg exercises
    Tubes/drain placement
    NPO/diet restrictions
    Bed rest

Postoperative Period
Collaborative Problems

Potential Complications
  Urinary retention
  Hemorrhage
  Hypovolemia/shock
  Renal failure
  Pneumonia (stasis)

  Thrombophlebitis
  Paralytic ileus
  Evisceration
  Dehiscence

Nursing Diagnoses

Potential for Infection: Wound, related to destruction of
  first line of defense against bacterial invasion
Potential Alteration in Respiratory Function related to
  postanesthesia state, postoperative immobility, and
  pain
Altered Comfort: Pain, related to surgical intervention
Activity Intolerance related to pain and fatigue
Self-care Deficits: (specify), related to limited mobility and
  pain
Potential Alteration in Bowel Elimination: Constipation,
  related to decreased peristalsis secondary to the
  effects of anesthesia, immobility, and pain
  medication
Alteration in Nutrition: Less Than Body Requirements,
  related to increased protein/vitamin requirements for
  wound healing and decreased intake secondary to
  pain, nausea, vomiting, and diet restrictions
Knowledge Deficit: (specify)
  Examples
    Home care
    Incisional care
    Signs and symptoms of
      complications

    Activity restriction
    Follow-up care

ABDOMINOPERINEAL RESECTION
(Colostomy, Ileostomy)

See also Cancer (General).
See also Surgery (General).

Preoperative Period
Nursing Diagnoses

Knowledge Deficit: (specify)
  Examples
    Stoma (appearance, care, site)
    Postoperative care

Postoperative Period
Nursing Diagnoses

Potential for Infection: Wound, related to fecal
    contamination
Disturbance in Self-concept related to effects of ostomy
    on self and relationship with others
Possible Sexual Dysfunction (Male) related to
    impotence secondary to surgical disruption of
    perineal structures
Potential Altered Sexualilty Patterns related to altered
    self-concept and change in appearance
Potential Social Isolation related to fear of loss of
    colostomy control, accident, or odor
Grieving (Client, Family) related to the implications of
    cancer and change in body functions
Knowledge Deficit: (specify)
  Examples
    Condition   Perineal wound care
    Skin care   Community
    Irritations   resources
    Odor control   (United Ostomy
    Signs and symptoms   Association)
        of complications

AMPUTATION

See Surgery (General).

Postoperative Period
Collaborative Problems
Potential Complications
    Edema   Infection

Hemorrhage　　　　　　　　*Contractures/muscle
atrophy*

Nursing Diagnoses

Grieving related to loss of limb or its effects on life-style

Impaired Home Maintenance Management related to
architectural barriers

Altered Comfort: Pain, related to surgical amputation or
phantom pain

Potential Disturbance in Self-concept related to loss of
body part

Fear related to surgical procedure, disability and resultant
change in life-style

Potential Alteration in Family Process related to change
in life-style (role responsibilities, financial,
occupational)

Impaired Physical Mobility related to altered gait

Potential for Injury related to altered gait or improper use
or fit of assistive devices

Impaired Adjustment related to (specify)

Knowledge Deficit: (specify)

    Examples

        Wound care

        Exercises

        Gait training

        Prosthesis

            Use

            Maintenance

            Position

ANEURYSM RESECTION (Abdominal Aortic)

See Surgery (General).

Postoperative Period
Collaborative Problems

Potential Complications
    *Cardiocirculatory (hypotension/hypertension, increased
cardiac workload, arrhythmias, electrolyte
imbalance, thrombus/embolus formation,
hemorrhage, compartmental syndrome,
thrombophlebitis)*
    *Graft (constriction, occlusion, disruption of anastomosis,
arterial spasm)*

Renal insufficiency
Paralytic ileus

Nursing Diagnoses

Alteration in Family Processes related to disruption of
family life, fear of outcome (death, disability), and
stressful environment (intensive care unit)
Knowledge Deficit: (specify)
  Examples
    Home care   Wound care
    Follow-up care

ANORECTAL SURGERY

See also Surgery (General).

Preoperative Period (see Hemorrhoids
or Anal Fissure)

Postoperative Period

Potential Complications
  Hemorrhage
  Urinary retention

Nursing Diagnoses

Altered Comfort: Pain, related to surgical incision and
spasms (sphincter, muscle)
Potential Alteration in Bowel Elimination: Constipation,
related to failure to respond to cues for defecation for
fear of pain
Potential for Infection: Anal Area, related to surgical
incision and fecal contamination
Knowledge Deficit: (specify)
  Examples
    Wound care
    Prevention of recurrence
    Nutritional requirements
      Diet
      Fluid
    Exercise program
    Signs and symptoms of complications

ARTERIAL BYPASS GRAFT OF LOWER EXTREMITY

(Aortic Iliac, Femoral, Popliteal)

See also Surgery (General).
See also Anticoagulant Therapy.

Postoperative Period
Collaborative Problems
Potential Complications
    Infection
    Occlusion of vessel

Disruption of
    anastomosis
    Hemorrhage

Nursing Diagnoses
Altered Comfort: Acute Pain, related to increased tissue
    perfusion to previous ischemic tissue
Knowledge Deficit: (specify)
  Examples
    Risk factors
    Foot care
    Incision care
    Signs of complications
    Follow-up care
    Implications of anticoagulant therapy
    Medications
    Activity restrictions

ARTHROPLASTY (Total Hip, Knee, or Ankle Replacement)

Preoperative Period
See also Surgery (General).
  Knowledge Deficit: Use of Trapeze

Postoperative Period
Potential Complications
    Fat emboli
    Hematoma formation
    Infection
    Dislocation of joint

    Stress fractures
    Neurovascular alterations
    Synovial herniation
    Thromboemboli formation

Nursing Diagnoses
Potential Impairment of Skin Integrity related to
    immobility and incision
Activity Intolerance related to fatigue, pain, and impaired
    gait
Impaired Home Maintenance Management related to
    postoperative flexion restrictions

Potential Alteration in Bowel Elimination: Constipation, related to activity restriction

Potential for Injury related to altered gait and assistive devices

Knowledge Deficit: (specify)
  Examples
    Activity restrictions
    Use of supportive devices
      Walker
      Crutches
      Canes
    Rehabilitative program
    Follow-up care
    Apparel restrictions
    Signs of complications
    Follow-up care
    Supportive services
    Prevention of infection

ARTHROSCOPY, ARTHROTOMY, MENISCECTOMY, BUNIONECTOMY

See also Surgery (General).

Preoperative Period

Knowledge Deficit: Crutch-walking and Leg Exercises

Postoperative Period
Collaborative Problems

Potential Complications
  Hematoma formation   *Hemorrhage*
  Neurovascular   *Effusion*
    impairments

Nursing Diagnoses

Knowledge Deficit: (specify)
  Examples
    Home care
    Incision care
    Activity restrictions
    Signs of complications
    Follow-up care

CAROTID ENDARTERECTOMY

See also Surgery (General).

Postoperative Period
Collaborative Problems

Potential Complications
  *Circulatory (cerebrovascular accident, hemorrhage,
      hypovolemia/hypervolemia, thrombus/embolus
      formation)*
  Tracheal deviation
  Laryngeal edema
  Cranial nerve impairment (VII, X, XI, XII)

Nursing Diagnoses

Potential for Injury related to syncope
Knowledge Deficit: (specify)
  Examples
    Risk factors
      Smoking
      Diet
      Obesity
    Activity restrictions
    Surgical site care
    Signs of complications
    Follow-up care

CESAREAN SECTION

See General Surgery.
See Postpartum Period.

CHOLECYSTECTOMY

See also Surgery (General).

Preoperative Period
Collaborative Problems

Potential Complications
  Peritonitis

Nursing Diagnoses

Potential Alteration in Respiratory Function related to
    high abdominal incision and splinting secondary to
    pain

Potential Alteration in Oral Mucous Membrane related to
NPO state and mouth breathing secondary to
nasogastric intubation

CRANIAL SURGERY

See also Surgery (General).
See also Brain Tumor for preoperative/postoperative care.
Potential Complications
  *Increased intracranial
    pressure*
  Seizures
  Respiratory insufficiency
  *Hypotension/
    hypertension*
  *Fluid/electrolyte
    imbalances*

  *Cranial nerve dysfunction
    (infratentorial)*
  *Cardiac dysrhythmias
    (infratentorial)*
  Gastrointestinal bleeding
  Meningitis/encephalitis

DILATATION AND CURETTAGE (D&C)

See also Surgery (General; preoperative and postoperative).

Postoperative Period
Collaborative Problems
Potential Complications
  Hemorrhage

Nursing Diagnoses
Knowledge Deficit: (specify)
  Examples
    Condition
    Home care

    Signs and symptoms of
      complications
    Activity restrictions

FRACTURED HIP

See also Surgery (General).

Preoperative Period
Nursing Diagnoses
Altered Comfort: Pain, related to trauma and muscle
  spasms
Knowledge Deficit: Use of Trapeze

Postoperative Period
Collaborative Problems
Potential Complications
  Dislocation of hip joint   Avascular necrosis of
                                             femoral head

Nursing Diagnoses
Self-care Deficit: (specify), related to activity restrictions
Knowledge Deficit: (specify)
  Examples
    Exercises
    Activity restrictions
    Home care
    Surgical site care
    Follow-up care
    Supportive services
    Ambulation assistance devices
      Crutches
      Walker

HYSTERECTOMY (Vaginal, Abdominal)

See also Surgery (General).

Postoperative Period
Collaborative Problems
Potential Complications
  Vaginal bleeding (post-   Fistula formation
      packing removal)   Deep vein thrombosis
  Urinary retention (post-   Trauma (ureter, bladder,
      catheter removal)   rectum)

Nursing Diagnoses
Potential for Infection related to surgical intervention and
    urinary catheter
Potential Disturbance in Self-concept related to
    implications of loss of body part
Potential Altered Sexuality Patterns related to personal
    significance of loss of body part and implications of
    loss on life-style
Grieving related to loss of body part and childbearing
    ability

Knowledge Deficit: (specify)
   Examples
      Perineal/incisional care
      Signs of complications
      Activity restrictions
        Sexual
        Activities of daily living
        Occupational
      Loss of menses
      Follow-up care (routine gynecological exams)

LAMINECTOMY

See also Surgery (General).

Preoperative Period
Nursing Diagnoses

Anxiety/Fear related to possibility of postoperative
    paralysis
Knowledge Deficit: (specify)
   Examples
      Postoperative care   Monitoring
      Positioning   Logrolling

Postoperative Period
Collaborative Problems

Potential Complications
  Neurosensory impairments
  Bowel/bladder dysfunction
  Cord edema
  Skeletal misalignment
  Cerebrospinal fluid leakage
  Hematoma

Nursing Diagnoses

Potential for Injury related to vertigo secondary to
    postural hypotension
Altered Comfort: Pain, related to muscle spasms (back,
    thigh) secondary to irritation of nerves during surgery
Impaired Physical Mobility related to treatment
    restrictions
Potential Diversional Activity Deficit related to monotony
    of immobility

Self-care Deficit: (specify), related to activity restrictions
Knowledge Deficit: (specify)
    Examples
        Activity restrictions   Exercises
        Immobilization device

MASTECTOMY

See also Cancer (General).
See also Surgery (General).

Preoperative Period
Nursing Diagnoses

Fear related to diagnosis of cancer and future
    implications

Postoperative Period
Collaborative Problems

Potential Complications
  Edema formation   *Neurovascular deficits*
Potential Fluid Volume Excess related to lymphedema
    secondary to surgical intervention
Self-care Deficit: (specify), related to impaired mobility of
    upper limb and limited range of motion
Potential for Injury related to vascular, lymphatic
    alteration of upper limb
Disturbance in Self-concept related to loss of body part
    (breast) and lymphedema
Potential Altered Sexuality Patterns related to loss of body
    part and fear of response of partner
Potential Social Isolation related to edema formation and
    fear of response of others
Knowledge Deficit: (specify)
    Examples
        Condition
        Home care
          Arm exercises
          Wound care
        Breast self-examination
        Hazards to affected arm
          Injections
          Pressure

Community services
Reach for Recovery
Apparel

MYOCARDIAL REVASCULARIZATION
(Coronary Artery Bypass)

See also Surgery (General).
See also Mechanical Ventilation.
See also Thoracic Surgery.

Postoperative Period
Collaborative Problems

Potential Complications
Death
Dysrhythmia (ventricular,
rate, junctional)
Hypertension/
hypotension
Hemorrhage
Vasodilatation
Myocardial infarction
(perioperative)
Low cardiac output
syndrome
Cardiac tamponade
Respiratory failure
Pulmonary embolism
Renal failure
Cerebrovascular accident
(embolus/thrombus)
Hypovolemia

Nursing Diagnoses

Altered Comfort: Acute Pain, related to surgical incisions,
drainage tube, and invasive catheters

Anxiety/Fear related to intensive environment of critical
care unit and potential for complications

Impaired Verbal Communication related to endotracheal
intubation (temporary)

Sleep Pattern Disturbance related to interruptions (noise,
treatments, activity)

Potential Alteration in Self-concept related to symbolic
meaning of heart and change in life-style

Alteration in Family Processes related to disruption of
family life, fear of outcome (death, disability), and
stressful environment (intensive care unit [ICU])

Knowledge Deficit: (specify)
Examples
Condition
Pain management
Angina
Incisional

Incisional care
Risk factors
  Smoking
  Diet
  Obesity
Restrictions
  Activity
  Sexual
Stress management techniques
Signs and symptoms of complications
Follow-up care
Pharmacologic care
Nutritional therapy
Exercise program

OPHTHALMIC SURGERY

See also Surgery (General).

Preoperative Period
Nursing Diagnoses

Knowledge Deficit:
  Examples
    Postoperative positioning
    Postoperative eye care/bandaging
    Postoperative activity restrictions
      Positioning
      Bending
      Stooping
      Straining
Fear/Anxiety related to having surgery with a local
  anesthetic, possible loss of vision, and fear of pain
  during procedure
Potential for Injury related to impaired vision and
  unfamiliar environment

Postoperative Period
Collaborative Problems

Potential Complications
  Swelling   Increased pain
  Eye damage   Change in vision

Nursing Diagnoses

Potential for Injury related to impaired vision and unfamiliar environment

Disturbance in Self-concept related to altered appearance secondary to surgery

Diversional Activity Deficits related to inability to participate in recreational activities secondary to impaired vision

Potential Social Isolation related to fear of embarrassment

Knowledge Deficit: (specify)

  Examples

    Activity restriction

      Coughing

      Eye movements

      Stooping

      Straining

      Bending

      Swimming

      Lifting heavy objects

    Eye care

    Signs and symptoms of complications

    Pharmacologic therapy

OTIC SURGERY (Stapedectomy, Tympanoplasty, Myringotomy, Tympanic Mastoidectomy)

See also General Surgical Plan.

Preoperative Period
Nursing Diagnosis

Anxiety/Fear related to possibility of greater loss of hearing after surgery

Postoperative Period
Collaborative Problems

Potential Complications

  Hemorrhage   Infection

  Facial paralysis   Impaired hearing/
                            deafness

Nursing Diagnoses

Impaired Communication related to decreased hearing

Potential Social Isolation related to embarrassment of not being able to hear in a social setting

Potential for Injury related to vertigo
Knowledge Deficit: (specify)
  Examples
    Signs and symptoms of complications
      Facial nerve injury
      Vertigo
      Tinnitus
      Gait disturbances
      Ear discharge
    Ear care
    Contradictions
      Swimming
      Shampooing
      Air flights
      Showering
      Nose blowing
      Sneezing
      Coughing
      Straining
    Follow-up care

PELVIC EXENTERATION

See also Cancer (General).
See also Surgery (General).
See also Abdominal–Perineal Resection (Total).

Preoperative Period
Nursing Diagnosis
  Knowledge Deficit
    Procedure
    Postoperative care

Postoperative Period
Collaborative Problems
Potential Complications
  Sepsis   Urinary stasis
  Paralytic ileus

Nursing Diagnoses
Altered Comfort: Pain, related to surgical intervention
    and metastasis
Grieving related to loss of body parts and function and
    effects on life-style and relationships

Fear related to possibility of recurrence of cancer

Potential Sexual Dysfunction related to
> Examples
>> Altered sexual function
>> Feelings of being undesirable
>> Partner's negative response (actual or perceived)
>> Physiological limitations

Potential Impaired Home Maintenance Management related to effects of debilitating disease and surgery on ability to maintain home

Self-care Deficit: (specify), related to pain, fatigue, and decreased motivation secondary to depression

Alteration in Family Processes related to effects of hospitalization, disease process, surgical intervention, and fears of recurrence on relationships and ability to meet role responsibilities

Potential Hopelessness related to nature of condition and its implications

Knowledge Deficit: (specify)
> Examples

Signs and symptoms of complications	Home care
	Community services
Pharmacologic therapy	

RADICAL NECK DISSECTION (Laryngectomy)

Preoperative Period
See also Surgery (General).
See also Cancer (General).

Nursing Diagnoses
Anxiety related to impending surgery and implications of condition on life-style

Knowledge Deficit: (specify)
> Examples
>> Postoperative disposition (intensive care unit)
>> Ability to communicate
>>> Reading
>>> Writing
>> Tracheostomy

Postoperative Period
Collaborative Problems
Potential Complications

Hypoxia	Tracheal edema

Carotid rupture   Cranial nerve injury
Hemorrhage   Infection

Nursing Diagnoses

Ineffective Airway Clearance related to increased
    secretions secondary to tracheostomy
Potential for Infection: Tracheostomy Site, related to
    excessive pooling of secretions and bypassing of
    upper respiratory defenses
Potential Impaired Physical Mobility: Shoulder and Neck
    related to muscle trauma secondary to surgery
Alteration in Oral Mucous Membrane related to excessive
    secretions or xerostomia
Impaired Verbal Communication related to inability to
    speak secondary to tracheostomy
Alteration in Self-concept related to disfiguring surgery
    and response of others to disfigurement
Potential Altered Sexuality Patterns related to change in
    appearance and responses of others to condition
Sensory–Perceptual Alterations: Olfactory, related to
    neural–sensory deficits secondary to surgery
Impaired Swallowing related to effects of surgery
Grieving related to loss of voice, olfactory sense, and
    previous appearance
Knowledge Deficit: (specify)
    Examples
        Condition
        Home care
            Oral hygiene
            Suctioning techniques
            Tracheostomy care
            Humidification
        Contraindications (lifting)
        Signs and symptoms of complications
            Swelling
            Pain
            Difficulty swallowing
            Purulent sputum
        Follow-up care
        Identificiation card/medallion
        Esophageal breathing
        Community services (American Cancer Society)

RENAL SURGERY (General, Percutaneous Nephrostomy/Extracorporeal Renal Surgery, Nephrectomy)

See also Surgery (General).

Collaborative Problems

Potential Complications
   Hemorrhage
   Shock
   Paralytic ileus
   Pneumothorax
   Of nephrostomy tube (calculi, fistulae, kinks)
Altered Comfort: Acute Pain, related to distention of
      renal capsule and incision
Potential Alteration of Respiratory Function related to
      pain on breathing and coughing secondary to
      location of incision
Knowledge Deficit: (specify)
   Examples
      Nephrostomy care
      Signs and symptoms of complications

RENAL TRANSPLANT

See also Corticosteroid Therapy.
See also Surgery (General).

Collaborative Problems

Potential Complications
   Hemodynamic instability
   Hypervolemia/hypovolemia
   Hypertension/hypotension
   Renal failure (donor kidney)
      Examples
         Ischemic damage prior to implantation
         Hematoma
         Rupture of anastomosis
         Bleeding at anastomosis
         Renal vein thrombosis
         Renal artery stenosis
         Blockage of ureter (kinks, clots)
         Kinking of ureter, renal artery
   Rejection of donor tissue

Excessive immunosuppression
Electrolyte imbalances (potassium, phosphate)
Deep vein thrombosis
Sepsis

Nursing Diagnoses

Potential for Infection related to altered immune system
secondary to medications

Potential Alteration in Oral Mucous Membrane related to
increased susceptibility to infection secondary to
immunosuppression

Potential Disturbance in Self-concept related to transplant
experience and potential for rejection

Fear related to possibility of rejection and dying

Potential Noncompliance related to complexity of
treatment regimen (diet, medications, record-keeping,
weight, blood pressure, urine testing) and euphoria
(post-transplant)

Knowledge Deficit: (specify)
  Examples
    Prevention of infection
    Personal hygiene
    Wound care
    Avoidance of contagious agents
  Activity progression
  Dietary management
  Daily recording
    Intake
    Output
    Weights
    Urine testing
    Blood pressure
    Temperature
  Pharmacologic therapy
    Purpose
    Timing
    Dosage
    Precautionary measures
    Potential adverse effects
  Daily urine testing (protein)
  Signs/symptoms of rejection/infection
  Avoidance of pregnancy
  Follow-up care
  Community resources

THORACIC SURGERY

See also Surgery (General).
See also Mechanical Ventilation.

Preoperative Period
Nursing Diagnoses

Anxiety/Fear related to possible respiratory difficulty
    after surgery
Knowledge Deficit: (specify)
    Examples
        Drainage devices
        Mechanical ventilation

Postoperative Period
Collaborative Problems

Potential Complications

Atelectasis	Hemorrhage
Pneumonia	Pulmonary embolus
Respiratory insufficiency	Subcutaneous
Complications of chest	emphysema
drainage	Mediastinal shift
Pneumothorax	

Nursing Diagnoses

Ineffective Airway Clearance related to difficulty in
    coughing secondary to pain
Altered Comfort: Acute Pain, related to surgical
    intervention and drainage tube(s)
Activity Intolerance related to reduction in exercise
    capacity secondary to loss of alveolar ventilation
Impaired Physical Mobility: Arm/Shoulder, related to
    muscle trauma secondary to surgery and position
    restrictions
Knowledge Deficit: (specify)
    Examples
        Condition
        Pain management
        Shoulder/arm exercises
        Incisional care
        Breathing exercises
        Splinting
        Environmental hazards
            Dust
            Smoke

Irritating chemicals
Crowds during epidemics of upper respiratory
    infection
Prevention of infection
Nutritional needs
Rest versus activity
Respiratory toilet
Follow-up care

TONSILLECTOMY

See also Surgery (General).

Collaborative Problems

Potential Complications
  Airway obstruction   *Aspiration*
  Hemorrhage

Nursing Diagnoses

Potential Fluid Volume Deficit related to decreased fluid
    intake secondary to pain on swallowing
Potential Alteration in Nutrition: Less Than Body
    Requirements, related to decreased intake secondary
    to pain on swallowing
Knowledge Deficit: (specify)
  Examples
    Rest requirements
    Nutritional needs
      Soft foods
      Fluids
    Signs and symptoms of complications (hemorrhage)
    Pain management
    Positioning
    Activity restrictions

TRANSURETHRAL RESECTION (Prostate
[Benign Hypertrophy or Cancer], Bladder Tumor)

See also Surgery (General).

Preoperative Period
Nursing Diagnoses

Knowledge Deficit: (specify)
  Examples
    Postoperative procedures
      Foley catheter

Murphy irrigation
Nephrostomy/pyelostomy tubes
Activity restrictions

Postoperative Period
Collaborative Problems

Potential Complications
Oliguria/anuria
Hemorrhage
Perforated bladder
(intraoperative)

Sepsis
Occlusion of drainage
devices

Nursing Diagnoses

Altered Comfort: Acute Pain, related to bladder spasms or
clots
Potential Altered Sexuality Patterns related to fear of
impotence resulting from surgical intervention
Knowledge Deficit: (specify)
Examples
Fluid requirements
Activity restrictions
Follow-up care

URINARY DIVERSION (Ileal Conduit, Ureterosigmoidostomy, Cutaneous Ureterostomy, Suprapubic Cystostomy)

See also Surgery (General).

Preoperative Period
Nursing Diagnoses

Anxiety/Fear related to
Examples
Surgical procedure
Diagnosis of cancer
Permanent loss of usual toilet habits
Effects on relationships
Management difficulties
Knowledge Deficit: (specify)
Examples
Procedure
Appliances

Postoperative Period
Collaborative Problems

Potential Complications

Urinary stasis	Stomal stenosis
Pyelonephritis	Renal calculi
Ureteral obstruction	

Nursing Diagnoses

Potential Impairment of Skin Integrity related to urine irritation around stoma

Potential Sexual Dysfunction related to effects of surgery on desire or ability to have sexual activity

Grieving related to loss of usual method of toileting and effects on life-style

Potential Disturbance in Self-concept related to effects of loss of body parts/function on life-style and relationships

Knowledge Deficit: (specify)

  Examples

    Condition

    Signs and symptoms of complications

    Nutritional therapy

    Fluid requirements

    Stoma care

    Odor control

    Appliance care

    Community services

Obstetric/Gynecologic Conditions

Obstetric Conditions

PRENATAL PERIOD (General)

Nursing Diagnoses

Altered Comfort: Nausea/Vomiting, related to elevated estrogen levels, decreased blood sugar or decreased gastric motility

Altered Comfort: Heartburn, related to pressure on cardiac sphincter from enlarged uterus

Alteration in Bowel Elimination: Constipation, related to decreased gastric motility and pressure of uterus on the lower colon

Activity Intolerance related to fatigue and dyspnea secondary to pressure of enlarging uterus on diaphragm and increased blood volume

Potential Alteration in Oral Mucous Membranes related to hyperemic gums secondary to estrogen and progesterone levels

Fear related to the possibility of having an imperfect baby

Potential for Infection: Vaginal, related to increased vaginal secretions secondary to hormonal changes

Potential for Injury related to syncope/hypotension secondary to peripheral venous pooling

Alteration in Comfort: Headaches, related to increased blood volume

Alteration in Comfort: Hemorrhoids, related to constipation and increased pressure of the enlarging uterus

Potential Disturbance in Self-concept related to effects of pregnancy on biopsychosocial patterns

Potential Alteration in Parenting (mother, father) related to

  Examples

    Knowledge deficit   Powerlessness

    Unwanted pregnancy   Feelings of
                                incompetency

Knowledge Deficit: (Specify)

  Examples

  Effects of pregnancy on

    Body systems

      Cardiovascular

      Integumentary

      Gastrointestinal

      Urinary

      Pulmonary

      Musculoskeletal

    Psychosocial domain

    Sexuality/sexual function

Family unit
    Spouse
    Children
Fetal growth and development
Nutritional requirements
Hazards of
    Smoking
    Excessive alcohol intake
    Drug abuse
    Excessive caffeine intake
    Excessive weight gain
Signs and symptoms of complications:
    Vaginal bleeding
    Cramping
    Gestational diabetes
    Excessive edema
    Preeclampsia
Preparation for childbirth
    Classes
    Printed references

ABORTION, INDUCED

Preprocedure Period
Nursing Diagnoses
Knowledge Deficit: (specify)
    Examples
        Options available
        Procedure
        Postprocedure care
        Normalcy of emotions

Postprocedure Period
Potential Ineffective Individual Coping: Depression,
        related to unresolved emotional responses (guilt) to
        societal, moral, religious, and familial opposition
Potential Alteration in Family Processes related to
        effects of procedure on relationships (disagreement
        regarding decisions, previous conflicts [personal,
        marital], or adolescent identity problems)

Knowledge Deficit: (specify)
  Examples
    Self-care
      Hygiene
      Breast care
    Nutritional needs
    Expected bleeding, cramping
    Signs and symptoms of complications
    Resumption of sexual activity
    Contraception
    Sex education as indicated
    Comfort measures
    Expected emotional responses
    Follow-up appointment
    Community resources

ABORTION, SPONTANEOUS

Nursing Diagnoses

Fear related to possibility of subsequent abortions
Grieving related to loss of pregnancy

EXTRAUTERINE PREGNANCY

(Ectopic Pregnancy)

Collaborative Problems

Potential Complications
  Hemorrhage   *Sepsis*
  Shock

Nursing Diagnoses

Grieving related to loss of fetus
Fear related to possibility of not being able to carry
    subsequent pregnancies
Altered Comfort: Pain, related to rupture of fallopian tube

HYPEREMESIS GRAVIDARUM

Collaborative Problems

Potential Complications
  Dehydration
  Negative nitrogen balance

Nursing Diagnoses

Potential Alteration in Nutrition: Less Than Body
    Requirements, related to vomiting

Anxiety related to ambivalent feeling toward pregnancy
    and parenthood

TOXEMIA

See also Prenatal Period.
See also Postpartum Period.
Potential Complications

Hypertension	Proteinuria
Seizures	Visual disturbances
Coma	Cerebral edema
Renal failure	Fetal compromise

Nursing Diagnoses

Activity Intolerance related to compromised oxygen
    supply

Anxiety/Fear related to the effects of condition on self,
    pregnancy, and infant

Potential Impairment of Skin Integrity related to
    generalized edema

Fluid Volume Excess: Edema, related to retention of
    water and impairment of sodium excretion secondary
    to impaired renal function

Potential for Injury related to vertigo, visual disturbances,
    or seizures

Knowledge Deficit: (specify)
    Examples

Dietary restrictions	Pharmacologic therapy
Signs and symptoms of complications	Comfort measures (headaches, backaches)
Conservation of energy	

UTERINE BLEEDING DURING PREGNANCY
(Placenta Previa, Abruptio Placentae,
Uterine Rupture, Nonmalignant
Lesions, Hydatidiform Mole)

See also Postpartum Period.

Collaborative Problems

Potential Complications

Hemorrhage	Renal failure
Shock	Fetal death
Disseminated	Anemia
intravascular	Sepsis
coagulation	

Nursing Diagnoses

Anxiety/Fear related to effects of bleeding on pregnancy and infant

Activity Intolerance related to the increased bleeding in response to activity

Grieving related to anticipated loss of pregnancy and loss of expected child

Fear related to possibility of subsequent future complications of pregnancy

INTRAPARTUM PERIOD (General)

Potential Complications

Hemorrhage (placenta	Fetal distress
previa, abruptio	Hypertension
placentae)	Uterine rupture

Altered Comfort related to uterine contractions during labor

Fear related to unpredictability of uterine contractions and possibility of having an impaired baby

Knowledge Deficit:

Examples

Relaxation/breathing exercises

Positioning

Procedures

Preparations (bowel, skin)

Frequent assessments

Anesthesia (regional, inhalation)

POSTPARTUM PERIOD (General, Mastitis [Lactational], Fetal/Newborn Death)

General Postpartum Period
Collaborative Problems

Potential Complications

Hemorrhage	Retained placental
Uterine atony	fragments

Lacerations   *Urinary retention*
Hematomas

Nursing Diagnoses

Potential for Infection: Vaginal, Perineal, related to
    bacterial invasion secondary to trauma during labor
    and delivery and episiotomy
Potential for Infection: breast related to milk production,
    and trauma during breastfeeding
Altered Comfort: Pain related to
    Examples
        Trauma to perineum   Hemorrhoids
            during labor and   Engorged breasts
            delivery   Involution of uterus
Potential Alteration in Bowel Elimination: Constipation,
    related to decreased intestinal peristalsis
    (postdelivery) and decreased activity
Potential Alteration in Parenting related to
    Examples
        Inexperience   Unwanted child
        Feelings of   Disappointment with
            incompetency   child
        Powerlessness   Lack of role models
Stress Incontinence related to tissue trauma during
    delivery
Potential Sleep Pattern Disturbance related to maternity
    department's routines and demands of newborn
Potential Disturbance in Self-concept related to body
    changes that persist postdelivery (skin, weight, and
    change in life-style)
Knowledge Deficit: (specify)
    Examples
        Postpartum routines
        Hygiene
            Breast
            Perineum
        Exercises
        Sexual counseling (contraception)
        Nutritional requirements (infant, maternal)
        Infant care
        Stresses of parenthood
        Adaptation of fathers
        Sibling relationships
        Parent/infant bonding

Postpartum emotional responses
Sleep/rest requirements
Household management
Community resources
Management of discomforts
Breast
Perineum
Social requirements
Mother
Couple
Signs and symptoms of complications

Mastitis (Lactational)
Collaborative Problems
Potential Complications
    Abscess

Nursing Diagnoses
Altered Comfort: Pain, related to inflammation of breast
    tissue
Knowledge Deficit: (specify)
    Examples
        Need for breast support
        Breast hygiene
        Breastfeeding restrictions
        Signs and symptoms of abscess formation

Fetal/Newborn Death
Nursing Diagnoses
Alteration in Family Processes related to emotional
    trauma of loss on each family member
Grieving related to loss of child
Fear related to the possibility of future fetal deaths

CONCOMITANT MEDICAL CONDITIONS
(Cardiac Disease [Prenatal, Postpartum], Diabetes
[Prenatal, Postpartum])

Cardiac Disease
See also Cardiac Disorders.
See also Prenatal Period.
See also Postpartum Period.

Collaborative Problems

Potential Complications

Congestive heart failure
Toxemia

Eclampsia
Valvular damage

Nursing Diagnoses

Anxiety/Fear related to effects of condition on self, pregnancy, and infant

Activity Intolerance related to increased metabolic requirements (pregnancy) in presence of compromised cardiac function

Impaired Home Maintenance Management related to impaired ability to perform role responsibilities during and after pregnancy

Potential Alteration in Family Processes related to disruption of activity restrictions and fears of effects on life-style

Knowledge Deficit: (specify)

Examples

Dietary requirements
(iron, protein)
Prevention of infection
Conservation of energy

Signs and symptoms of
complications
Community resources

Diabetes (Prenatal)

See also Prenatal Period.
See also Diabetes Mellitus.
See also Postpartum Period.

Collaborative Problems

Potential Complications

Hypoglycemia/
hyperglycemia
Hydramnios

Acidosis
Toxemia

Nursing Diagnoses

Potential Impairment of Skin Integrity related to excessive skin stretching secondary to hydramnios

Potential for Infection: Vaginal, related to susceptibility to monilial infection

Alteration in Comfort: Headaches, related to cerebral edema or hyperirritability

Knowledge Deficit: (specify)

Examples

Effects of pregnancy on diabetes

Effects of diabetes on pregnancy
Nutritional requirements
Insulin requirements
Signs and symptoms of complications
Frequent blood/urine samples

Diabetes (Postpartum)

See also Postpartum Period (General).
Collaborative Problems
Potential Complications
Hypoglycemia
Hyperglycemia
Toxemia
Eclampsia

Hemorrhage (secondary
to uterine atony from
excessive amniotic
fluid)

Nursing Diagnoses

Anxiety related to separation from infant secondary to the
need for special care needs of infant
Potential for Infection: Perineal Area related to depleted
host defenses and depressed leukocytic phagocytosis
secondary to hyperglycemia
Knowledge Deficit: (specify)
Examples
Risks of future pregnancies
Birth control methods
types contraindicated
Special care requirements for infant

Gynecologic Conditions

ENDOMETRIOSIS
Collaborative Problems
Potential Complications
Hypermenorrhea   Polymenorrhea

Nursing Diagnoses

Altered Comfort: Chronic Pain, related to response of
displaced endometrial tissue (abdominal, peritoneal)
to cyclic ovarian hormonal stimulation
Sexual Dysfunction related to painful intercourse or
infertility
Anxiety/Fear related to unpredictable nature of disease

Knowledge Deficit: (specify)
  Examples
    Condition   Pharmacologic therapy
    Myths   Potential for pregnancy

REPRODUCTIVE TRACT INFECTIONS (Vaginitis, Endometritis, Pelvic Cellulitis, Peritonitis)

Collaborative Problems

Potential Complications
  Septicemia   *Pneumonia*
  Abscess formation   *Pulmonary embolism*

Nursing Diagnoses

Altered Comfort: Pain, Chills, related to infectious process
Potential Fluid Volume Deficit related to inadequate
    intake, fatigue, pain, and fluid losses secondary to
    elevated temperature
Potential Ineffective Individual Coping: Depression,
    related to chronicity of condition and lack of
    definitive diagnosis/treatment
Potential Alteration in Body Temperature related to
    infectious process
Knowledge Deficit: (specify)
  Examples
    Condition   Signs and symptoms of
    Nutritional   recurrence/
      requirements   complications
                       Sleep/rest requirements

Neonatal Conditions

NEONATE, NORMAL

Collaborative Problems

Potential Complications
  Hypothermia
  Hypoglycemia

Hyperbilirubinemia
Bradycardia

Nursing Diagnoses

Potential for Infection (Nosocomial) related to
Vulnerability of infant
Lack of normal flora
Environmental hazards

Personnel	Open wounds
Other newborns	Umbilical cord
Parents	Circumcision

Potential Alteration in Respiratory Function related to oropharynx secretions

Potential Impairment of Skin Integrity related to susceptibility to nosocomial infection and lack of normal skin flora

Ineffective Thermoregulation related to newborn extrauterine transition

Knowledge Deficit (see Postpartum Period)

NEONATE, PREMATURE

See also Family of High-risk Neonate.

Collaborative Problems

Potential Complications

Cold stress	Hypocalcemia
Apnea	Sepsis
Bradycardia	Seizures
Hypoglycemia	Pneumonia
Acidosis	Hyperbilirubinemia

Nursing Diagnoses

Potential Alteration in Nutrition: Less Than Body Requirements related to diminished sucking

Potential Alteration in Bowel Elimination: Constipation related to decreased intestinal motility and immobility

Potential Alteration in Respiratory Function related to immobility and increased secretions

Potential for Infection (Nosocomial) related to
Vulnerability of infant
Lack of normal flora
Environmental hazards
Personnel

Other newborns
Parents
Open wounds
    Umbilical cord
    Circumcision
Potential Impairment of Skin Integrity related to
    susceptibility to nosocomial infection (lack of normal
    skin flora)
Ineffective Theromregulation related to newborn
    transition to extrauterine environment

NEONATE, POSTMATURE (Small for Gestational Age [SGA], Large for Gestational Age [LGA])

Collaborative Problems

Potential Complications
    Asphyxia at birth
    Meconium aspiration
    Hypoglycemia
    Polycythemia (SGA)
    Edema
        Generalized
        Cerebral
    Central nervous system depression
    Renal tubular necrosis
    Impaired intestinal absorption
    Birth injuries (LGA)

Nursing Diagnoses

Potential Impairment of Skin Integrity related to
    absence of protective vernix and prolonged
    exposure to amniotic fluid (LGA)
Potential Alteration in Nutrition: Less Than Body
    Requirements, related to swallowing difficulties

NEONATE WITH SPECIAL PROBLEM
(Congenital Infections—Cytomegalovirus [CMV], Rubella, Toxoplasmosis, Syphilis, Herpes)

See also High-risk Neonate.
See also Family of High-risk Neonate.
See also Developmental Problems/Needs under Pediatric Disorders.

Collaborative Problems

Potential Complications

Hyperbilirubinemia	Cataracts (rubella)
Hepatosplenomegaly	Retinitis
Anemia	Thrombocytopenic
Hydrocephalus	purpura (rubella)
Microcephaly	Sensory-motor deafness
Mental retardation	(CMV)
Congenital heart disease	Periostitis (syphilis)
(rubella)	Seizures

Nursing Diagnoses

Potential for Infection Transmission related to contagious nature of organism

Potential for Injury related to uncontrolled tonic/clonic movements

Potential Alteration in Nutrition: Less Than Body Requirements, related to poor sucking reflex

NEONATE OF A DIABETIC MOTHER

See also Neonate, Normal.
See also Family of High-risk Neonate.

Collaborative Problems

Potential Complications

Hypoglycemia	Acidosis
Hypocalcemia	Birth injury (macrosomia)
Polycythemia	Hyaline membrane
Hyperbilirubinemia	disease (if
Sepsis	premature)
Respiratory distress	Venous thrombosis
syndrome	

Nursing Diagnosis

Potential Fluid Volume Deficit related to increased urinary excretion and osmotic diuresis

HIGH-RISK NEONATE

See also Family of High-risk Neonate.

Collaborative Problems

Potential Complications

Anoxia	Seizures

Shock   *Hypotension*
Respiratory distress   *Septicemia*

Nursing Diagnoses

Altered Comfort related to abdominal distention

Potential Alteration in Nutrition: Less Than Body
    Requirements, related to poor sucking reflex
    secondary to (specify)

Potential for Injury related to uncontrolled tonic/clonic
    movements or hyperirritability

Potential for Infection (Nosocomial) related to
  Vulnerability of infant
  Lack of normal flora
  Environmental hazards
    Personnel
    Other newborns
    Parents
  Open wounds
    Umbilical cord
    Circumcision

Potential Alteration in Respiratory Function related to
    oropharyngeal secretions

Potential Impairment of Skin Integrity related to
    susceptibility to nosocomial infection secondary to
    lack of normal skin flora

Potential Alteration in Tissue Perfusion related to
    hypothermia

Ineffective Thermoregulation related to newborn
    transition to extrauterine environment

FAMILY OF HIGH-RISK NEONATE

Nursing Diagnoses

Grieving related to realization of present or future loss
    for family and/or child

Alteration in Family Processes related to effect of
    extended hospitalization on family (role
    responsibilities, finances)

Anxiety related to unpredictable prognosis

Potential Alteration in Parenting related to inadequate
    bonding secondary to parent–child separation or
    failure to accept impaired child

Ineffective Individual Coping: Depression, related to
    perceived parental role failure

HYPERBILIRUBINEMIA (Rh Incompatibility, ABO Incompatibility)

See also Family of High-risk Neonate.
See also Neonate, Normal.

Collaborative Problems

Potential Complications

Anemia
Jaundice
Kernicterus
Hepatosplenomegaly
Hydrops fetalis (cardiac
    failure, hypoxia,
    anasarca, and
    pericardial, pleural,
    and peritoneal
    effusions)

Renal failure
    (phototherapy
    complications,
    hyperthermia/
    hypothermia,
    dehydration,
    priapism, "bronze
    baby" syndrome)

Nursing Diagnoses

Potential Impaired Tissue Integrity: Cornea, related to
    exposure to phototherapy light and continuous
    wearing of eye pads
Potential Impairment of Skin Integrity related to diarrhea,
    urinary excretions of bilirubin, and exposure to
    phototherapy light

NEONATE OF NARCOTIC-ADDICTED MOTHER

See also Family of High-risk Neonate.
See also Neonate, Normal.
See also Substance Abuse for Mother.

Collaborative Problems

Potential Complications

Hyperirritability/seizures
Withdrawal
Hypocalcemia
Hypoglycemia

Sepsis
Dehydration
Electrolyte imbalances
Aspiration

Nursing Diagnoses

Potential Alteration in Nutrition: Less Than Body
    Requirements, related to uncoordinated and
    ineffective sucking and swallowing reflexes

Potential Impairment of Skin Integrity related to
  generalized diaphoresis and marked rigidity
Alteration in Bowel Elimination: Diarrhea, related to
  increased peristalsis secondary to hyperirritability
Sleep/Pattern Disturbance related to hyperirritability
Potential for Injury: Blisters, related to frantic sucking of
  fists
Potential for Injury related to uncontrolled tremors or
  tonic/clonic movements
Sensory–Perceptual Alterations related to hypersensitivity
  to environmental stimuli

RESPIRATORY DISTRESS SYNDROME

See also High-risk Neonate.
See also Mechanical Ventilation.

Collaborative Problems

Potential Complications
  Hypoxia   Sepsis
  Atelectasis   Hyperthermia
  Acidosis

Nursing Diagnoses

Activity Intolerance related to insufficient oxygenation of
  tissues secondary to impaired respirations
Potential for Infection (Nosocomial) related to
  vulnerability of infant, lack of normal flora,
  environmental hazards (personnel, other newborns,
  parents), and open wounds (umbilical cord,
  circumcision)
Potential Impairment of Skin Integrity related to
  susceptibility to nosocomial infection and lack of
  normal skin flora

SEPSIS (Septicemia)

See also Newborn.
See also Family of High-risk Neonate.

Collaborative Problems

Potential Complications
  Anemia   Seizures
  Respiratory distress Hepatosplenomegaly

Hypothermia/	*Hemorrhage*
hyperthermia	*Jaundice*
Hypotension	*Meningitis*
Edema	*Pyarthrosis*

Nursing Diagnoses

Potential Impairment of Skin Integrity related to edema
and immobility

Alteration in Nutrition: Less Than Body Requirements,
related to poor sucking reflex

Alteration in Bowel Elimination: Diarrhea, related to
intestinal irritation secondary to infecting organism

Potential for Injury related to uncontrolled tonic/clonic
movements

Potential for Injury: Ecchymosis, related to hematopoietic
insufficiency

Potential Alteration in Body Temperature related to body
response to pathogens

Pediatric/Adolescent Disorders*

DEVELOPMENTAL PROBLEMS/NEEDS RELATED TO CHRONIC ILLNESS
(*e.g.,* Permanent Disability, Multiple Handicaps, Developmental Disability [Mental/Physical], Life-threatening Illness)

Nursing Diagnoses

Grieving (Parental) related to anticipated losses
secondary to condition

For additional pediatric medical diagnoses, see the adult diagnoses and also Developmental Problems/Needs; for example:

Diabetes mellitus	Neoplastic disorders
Anorexia nervosa (psychiatric	Fractures
disorders)	Congestive heart failure
Spinal cord injury	Pneumonia
Head trauma	

Alteration in Family Processes related to adjustment
   requirements for situation
   Examples
      Time
      Energy
         Emotional
         Physical
      Financial
      Physical care
Potential Impaired Home Maintenance Management
   related to inadequate resources, housing, or
   impaired caregiver(s)
Potential Alterations in Parental Role related to
   separations secondary to frequent hospitalizations
Potential Social Isolation (Child/Family) related to the
   disability and the requirements of the caregiver(s)
Potential Alteration in Parenting related to abuse,
   rejection, overprotection secondary to inadequate
   resources or coping mechanisms
Anxiety (Parental) related to illness, health-care
   interventions, and parent–child separation
Self-care Deficit: (specify), related to illness limitations
   or hospitalization
Potential Altered Growth and Development related to
   impaired ability to achieve developmental tasks
   secondary to restrictions imposed by disease,
   disability, or treatments

ASTHMA

See also Developmental Problems/Needs.

Collaborative Problems

Potential Complications
   Hypoxia   *Respiratory acidosis*
   Corticosteroid therapy

Nursing Diagnoses

Ineffective Airway Clearance related to bronchospasm and
   increased pulmonary secretions
Fear related to breathlessness and recurrences
Potential Alteration in Respiratory Function related to
   increased pulmonary secretions

Knowledge Deficit: (specify)
  Examples
    Condition
    Environmental hazards
      Smoking
      Allergens
      Weather
    Prevention of infection
    Breathing/relaxation exercises
    Signs and symptoms of complications
    Pharmacologic therapy
    Fluid requirements
    Behavioral modification
    Daily diary recording

CELIAC DISEASE

See also Developmental Problems/Needs.

Collaborative Problems

Potential Complications

Severe malnutrition/ dehydration	*Electrolyte imbalances*
Anemia	*Metabolic acidosis*
Altered blood coagulation	*Shock*
Osteoporosis	*Delayed growth*

Nursing Diagnoses

Potential Alteration in Nutrition: Less Than Body
  Requirements, related to malabsorption, dietary
  restrictions, and anorexia
Alteration in Bowel Elimination: Diarrhea/Steatorrhea,
  related to decreased absorption in small intestines
  secondary to damaged villi resulting from toxins
  from undigested gliadin
Potential Fluid Volume Deficit related to fluid loss in
  diarrhea
Knowledge Deficit: (specify)
  Examples
    Dietary management
      Restrictions
      Vitamin

Protein
Carbohydrate requirements

CEREBRAL PALSY*

See also Developmental Problems/Needs.

Collaborative Problems

Potential Complications

Contractures   Respiratory infections
Seizures

Nursing Diagnoses

Potential for Injury related to inability to control
  movements
Potential Alteration in Nutrition: Less Than Body
  Requirements, related to sucking difficulties (infant)
  and dysphagia
Self-care Deficit (specify) related to sensory-motor
  impairments
Impaired Verbal Communication related to impaired
  ability to speak words related to facial muscle
  involvement
Potential Fluid Volume Deficit related to difficulty
  obtaining or swallowing liquids
Potential Diversional Activity Deficit related to effects of
  limitations on ability to participate in recreational
  activities
Knowledge Deficit: (specify)
  Examples
    Disease   Education
    Pharmacologic regime   Community services
    Activity program   Orthopedic appliances

CHILD ABUSE (Battered Child Syndrome,
Child Neglect)

See also Fractures, Burns.
See also Failure to Thrive.

---

* Because disabilities associated with cerebral palsy can be varied
(hemiparesis, quadriparesis, diplegia, monoplegeia, triplegia, paraplegia), the nurse will have to specify the child's limitations clearly
in the diagnostic statements.

Collaborative Problems

Potential Complications
Trauma (fractures, burns,
    lacerations)
Behavioral disorders
    (withdrawal,
    aggression)
Failure to thrive
Malnutrition

Vandalism
Drug or alcohol addiction
    (older child)
Venereal disease
Pregnancy in young
    adolescent

Nursing Diagnoses

Ineffective Family Coping related to presence of factors
    that contribute to child abuse:
    Examples
        Lack of or unavailability of extended family
        Economic conditions
            Inflation
            Unemployment
        Lack of role model as a child
        High-risk children
            Unwanted
            Of undesired gender or appearance
            Physically or mentally handicapped
            Hyperactive
            Terminally ill
        High-risk parents
            Single
            Adolescent
            Emotionally disturbed
            Alcoholic
            Drug-addicted
            Physically ill
Ineffective Individual Coping (Child Abuser) related to
    Examples
        History of abuse by own parents and lack of warmth
            and affection from them
        Social isolation (few friends or outlets for tensions)
        Marked lack of self-esteem, with low tolerance for
            criticism
        Emotional immaturity and dependency
        Distrust of others
        Inability to admit need for help

High expectations for/of child (perceiving child as a
source of emotional gratification)
Unrealistic desire for child to give pleasure
Ineffective Individual Coping (Nonabusing Parent) related
to passive and compliant response to abuse
Fear related to possibility of placement in a shelter or
foster home
Anxiety/Fear (Parental) related to responses of others
guilt, possible loss of child, and criminal prosecution
Potential Alteration in Nutrition: Less Than Body
Requirements, related to inadequate intake secondary
to lack of knowledge or neglect
Knowledge Deficit: (specify)
  Examples
    Parenting skills
      Discipline
      Expectations
    Constructive stress management
    Signs and symptoms of abuse
    High-risk groups
      Parent(s)
      Child
    Child protection laws
    Community services
      Hotlines
      Counselling

CLEFT LIP AND PALATE

See also Developmental Problems/Needs.
See also Surgery (General).

Preoperative Period
Nursing Diagnoses

Potential Alteration in Nutrition: Less Than Body
Requirements, related to inability to suck secondary
to cleft lip

Postoperative Period
Collaborative Problems

Potential Complications
  Respiratory distress   *Failure to thrive (organic)*

Nursing Diagnoses

Impaired Physical Mobility related to restricted activity secondary to use of restraints

Potential Impaired Verbal Communication related to impaired muscle development, insufficient palate function, faulty dentition, or hearing loss

Potential Ineffective Airway Clearance related to impaired sucking

Knowledge Deficit: (specify)

Examples

Condition

Feeding and suctioning techniques

Surgical site care

Risks for otis media (dental/oral problems)

Referral to speech therapist

COMMUNICABLE DISEASES

See also Developmental Problems/Needs.

Nursing Diagnoses

Altered Comfort related to fatigue, malaise, sore throat, elevated temperature

Potential for Infection Transmission related to contagious agents

Potential Fluid Volume Deficit related to increased fluid loss secondary to elevated temperature or insufficient oral intake secondary to malaise

Potential Alteration in Nutrition: Less Than Body Requirements, related to anorexia and sore throat or pain on chewing (mumps)

Altered Comfort: Photophobia, related to disorder

Altered Comfort: Pruritus, related to lesions

Potential Ineffective Airway Clearance related to increased mucus production (whooping cough)

Knowledge Deficit: (specify)

Examples

Condition   Immunizations

Transmission   Skin care

Prevention

CONVULSIVE DISORDERS

See also Developmental Problems/Needs.
See also Mental Disabilities, if indicated.

Collaborative Problems

Potential Complications
  Respiratory arrest
  Hypoxia

Nursing Diagnoses

Potential for Injury related to uncontrolled movements of
    seizure activity
Anxiety related to embarrassment and fear of seizure
    episodes
Potential Ineffective Individual Coping: Aggression,
    related to restrictions, parental overprotection,
    parental indulgence
Knowledge Deficit: (specify)
  Examples
    Condition/cause
    Pharmacologic therapy
    Treatment during seizures
    Seizure precautions
    Environmental hazards
      Water
      Driving
      Heights

CYSTIC FIBROSIS

See also Developmental Problems/Needs.

Collaborative Problems

Potential Complications
  Bronchopneumonia,   *Paralytic ileus*
    atelectasis

Nursing Diagnoses

Ineffective Airway Clearance related to mucopurulent
    secretions
Potential Alteration in Nutrition: Less Than Body
    Requirements, related to need for increased calories
    and protein secondary to impaired intestinal
    absorption, loss of fat, and fat-soluable vitamins in
    stools
Alteration in Bowel Elimination: Constipation/Diarrhea,
    related to excessive or insufficient pancreatic enzyme
    replacement

Activity Intolerance related to dyspnea secondary to
  mucopurulent secretions
Knowledge Deficit: (specify)
  Examples
    Condition (genetic transmission)
    Risk for infection
    Pharmacological therapy
      Side-effects
      Ototoxicity
      Renal toxicity
    Equipment
      Oxygen
      Nebulization
    Nutritional therapy
    Salt replacement requirements
    Breathing exercises
    Postural drainage
    Exercise program
    Community resources (Cystic Fibrosis Foundation)

DOWN SYNDROME

See also Developmental Problems/Needs.
See also Mental Disabilities, if indicated.

Nursing Diagnoses

Potential Alteration in Respiratory Function related to
  decreased respiratory expansion secondary to
  decreased muscle tone, inadequate mucus
  drainage, and mouth-breathing
Potential Impairment of Skin Integrity related to rough,
  dry skin surface and flaccid extremities
Potential Alteration in Bowel Elimination:
  Constipation, related to decreased gastric motility
Alteration in Nutrition: Less Than Body Requirements
  (Infant), related to sucking difficulties secondary to
  large, protruding tongue
Potential Alteration in Nutrition: Greater Than Body
  Requirements, related to increased caloric
  consumption secondary to boredom in the
  presence of limited physical activity
Self-care Deficits: (specify), related to physical
  limitations

Knowledge Deficit: (specify)
    Examples

Condition	Education
Home care	Community services

FAILURE TO THRIVE (Nonorganic)

See also Developmental Problems/Needs.

Collaborative Problems

Potential Complications

Metabolic dysfunction	Dehydration

Nursing Diagnoses

Ineffective Individual Coping (Caregiver) related to failure
    to respond to child's needs (emotional/physical)
    secondary to caregiver's emotional problems

Alteration in Nutrition: Less Than Body Requirements,
    related to inadequate intake secondary to the lack of
    emotional and sensory stimulation or lack of
    knowledge of caregiver

Sensory–Perceptual Alterations related to history of
    insufficient sensory input from primary caregiver

Sleep Pattern Disturbance related to anxiety and
    apprehension secondary to parental deprivation

Alteration in Parenting related to
    Examples

Lack of Knowledge of parenting skills	Relationship problems
Impaired caregiver	Unrealistic expectations for child
Impaired child	Unmet psychological needs
Lack of support system	
Lack of role model	

Impaired Home Maintenance Management related to
    difficulty of caregiver with maintaining a safe home
    environment

Knowledge Deficit: (specify)
    Examples

Growth and development requirements	Risk for child abuse
	Parenting skills
	Community agencies
Feeding guidelines	

GLOMERULAR DISORDERS (Glomerulonephritis: Acute, Chronic; Nephrotic Syndrome: Congenital, Secondary, Idiopathic)

See also Developmental Problems/Needs.
See also Corticosteroid Therapy.

Collaborative Problems

Potential Complications

Anasarca (generalized edema)
Hypertension
Azotemia
Septicemia

Malnutrition
Ascites
Pleural effusion
Hypoalbuminemia

Nursing Diagnoses

Potential for Infection related to increased susceptibility during edematous phase and lowered resistance secondary to corticosteroid therapy

Potential Impairment of Skin Integrity related to
Examples

Immobility
Lowered resistance

Edema
Frequent application of collection bags

Alteration in Nutrition: Less Than Body Requirements, related to dietary restrictions, anorexia secondary to fatigue, malaise, and pressure on abdominal structures (edema)

Activity Intolerance related to fatigue

Diversional Activity Deficit related to hospitalization and impaired ability to perform usual activities

Knowledge Deficit: (specify)
Examples
Condition
Etiology
Course
Treatments
Signs and symptoms of complications
Pharmacologic therapy
Nutritional/fluid requirements
Prevention of infection
Home care
Diet
Urine testing

Follow-up care
Community services

HEMOPHILIA

See also Developmental Problems/Needs.

Collaborative Problems

Potential Complications
  Hemorrhage

Nursing Diagnoses

Altered Comfort: Acute, Chronic Pain, related to joint
    swelling and limitations secondary to hemarthrosis
Potential Impaired Physical Mobility related to joint
    swelling and limitations secondary to hemarthrosis
Potential Alteration in Oral Mucous Membranes related
    to trauma from coarse food and insufficient dental
    hygiene
Knowledge Deficit: (specify)
  Examples
    Condition   Environmental hazards
    Contraindications (*e.g.,*   Emergency treatment to
      aspirin)   control bleeding
    Genetic transmission

INFECTIOUS MONONUCLEOSIS (Adolescent)

Collaborative Problems

Potential Complications
  Enlarged spleen
  Hepatic dysfunction

Nursing Diagnoses

Activity Intolerance related to fatigue secondary to
    infectious process
Altered Comfort: Acute Pain, related to sore throat and
    headaches
Alteration in Health Maintenance related to need for
    nutritional counseling and sleep requirements
Potential Alteration in Nutrition: Less Than Body
    Requirements, related to sore throat and malaise
Grieving related to restrictions of disease and treatments
    on life-style

Potential for Infection Transmission related to contagious
condition
Knowledge Deficit: (specify)
  Examples
    Condition
    Communicable nature
    Diet therapy
    Risks of alcohol ingestion (with hepatic dysfunction)
    Signs and symptoms of complications
      Hepatic
      Splenic
      Neurologic
      Hematologic
    Activity restrictions

LEGG-CALVÉ-PERTHES DISEASE

See also Developmental Problems/Needs.

Collaborative Problems

Potential Complications
  Permanent deformed femoral head

Nursing Diagnoses

Altered Comfort: Pain, related to joint dysfunction
Potential Impairment of Skin Integrity related to
    immobilization devices (casts, braces)
Self-care Deficits: (specify), related to pain and
    immobilization devices
Knowledge Deficit: (specify)
  Examples
    Disease
    Weight-bearing restrictions
    Application/maintenance of devices
    Pain management at home

LEUKEMIA

See also Chemotherapy.
See also Radiation Therapy
See also Cancer (General).
See also Developmental Problems/Needs.

Collaborative Problems

Potential Complications
  Hepatosplenomegaly

Increased intracranial edema
Metastasis (brain, lungs, kidneys, gastrointestinal tract,
*   spleen, liver)*
Hypermetabolism
Hemorrhage
Dehydration
Myelosupression

Nursing Diagnoses

Potential for Infection related to altered immune system
    secondary to leukemic process and side-effects of
    chemotherapeutic agents

Potential Social Isolation related to effects of disease and
    treatments on appearance and fear of embarrassment

Potential Altered Growth and Development related to
    impaired ability to achieve developmental tasks
    secondary to limitations of disease and treatments

MENINGITIS (Bacterial)

See also Developmental Problems/Needs.

Collaborative Problems

Potential Complications
*   Peripheral circulatory collapse*
*   Disseminated intravascular coagulation*
*   Increased intracranial pressure/hydrocephalus*
*   Visual/auditory nerve palsies*
*   Paresis (hemi-, quadri-)*
*   Subdural effusions*
*   Respiratory distress*
*   Seizures*
*   Fluid/electrolyte imbalances*

Nursing Diagnoses

Potential for Injury related to seizure activity secondary to
    infectious process

Altered Comfort related to nuchal rigidity, muscle aches,
    and immobility

Sensory–Perceptual Alteration: Visual, Auditory, related
    to increased sensitivity to external stimuli secondary
    to infectious process

Impaired Physical Mobility related to intravenous
    infusion, nuchal rigidity, and restraining devices

Potential Impairment of Skin Integrity related to
    immobility

Potential Alteration in Body Temperature related to
   infectious processes
Knowledge Deficit: (specify)
   Examples
      Condition   Diagnostic procedures
      Antibiotic therapy

MENINGOMYELOCELE

See also Developmental Problems/Needs.

Collaborative Problems

Potential Complications
   Hydrocephalus/shunt infections
   Increased intracranial pressure
   Urinary tract infections
Reflex Incontinence related to sensory-motor dysfunction
Potential for Infection related to vulnerability of
   meningomyelocele sac
Potential Impairment of Skin Integrity related to
   sensorimotor impairments and orthopedic appliances
Self-care Deficit: (specify), related to sensory-motor
   impairments
Potential for Injury: Fractures, Membrane tears, related to
   pathological condition
Impaired Physical Mobility related to lower limb
   impairments
Grieving (Parental) related to birth of infant with defects
Knowledge Deficit: (specify)
   Examples
      Condition   Self-catheterization
      Home care   Activity program
      Orthopedic appliances   Community services

MENTAL DISABILITIES

See Developmental Problems/Needs.

Nursing Diagnoses

   Self-care Deficit: (specify) related to sensorimotor
      deficits
   Impaired Communication related to impaired receptive
      skills or impaired expressive skills
   Potential Social Isolation (family, child) related to fear
      and embarrassment of child's behavior/appearance

Knowledge Deficits: (specify)
> Examples
>> Condition
>> Child's potential
>> Home care

Community services
Education

MUSCULAR DYSTROPHY (Duchenne)

See also Developmental Problems/Needs.

Collaborative Problems

Potential Complications
> Seizures
> Respiratory infections

Metabolic failure

Nursing Diagnoses

Potential for Injury related to inability to control
> movements

Potential Alteration in Nutrition: Less Than Body
> Requirements, related to sucking difficulties (infant)
> and dysphagia

Self-care Deficits: (specify), related to sensory-motor
> impairments

Impaired Verbal Communication related to impaired
> ability to speak words secondary to facial muscle
> involvement

Potential Impaired Physical Mobility related to muscle
> weakness

Potential Alteration in Nutrition: More Than Body
> Requirements, related to increased caloric
> consumption secondary to boredom in presence of
> decreased metabolic needs secondary to limited
> physical activity

Grieving (Parental) related to progressive, terminal nature
> of the disease

Impaired Swallowing related to sensory-motor deficits

Potential Hopelessness related to progressive nature of
> disease

Potential Diversional Activity Deficit related to effects of
> limitations on ability to participate in recreational
> activities

Knowledge Deficit: (specify)
> Examples
>> Disease
>> Pharmacologic regimen
>> Activity program

Education
Community services

OBESITY

See also Developmental Problems/Needs.

Nursing Diagnoses

Ineffective Individual Coping related to increased food consumption in response to stressors

Alteration in Health Maintenance related to the need for

Exercise program   Behavioral modification
Nutrition counseling

Disturbance in Self-concept related to feelings of self-degradation and response of others (peers, family, others) to obesity

Alteration in Family Processes related to responses to and effects of weight loss therapy on parent/child relationship

Potential Impaired Social Interaction related to inability to initiate and maintain relationships secondary to feelings of embarrassment and negative responses of others

Knowledge Deficit: (specify)
Examples
Condition
Etiology
Course
Risks
Therapies available
Destructive versus constructive eating patterns
Self-help groups

OSTEOMYELITIS

See also Developmental Problems/Needs.

Collaborative Problems

Potential Complications
Infective emboli
Side-effects of antibiotic therapy (hematologic, renal, hepatic)

Nursing Diagnoses

Altered Comfort related to swelling, hyperthermia, and infectious process of bone

Diversional Activity Deficit related to impaired mobility
   and long-term hospitalization
Potential Alteration in Nutrition: Less Than Body
   Requirements, related to anorexia secondary to
   infectious process
Potential Alteration in Bowel Elimination: Constipation,
   related to immobility
Potential Impairment of Skin Integrity related to
   mechanical irritation of cast/splint
Potential for Injury: Pathological Fractures related to
   disease process
Knowledge Deficit: (specify)
   Examples
      Condition   Signs and symptoms of
      Wound care   complications
      Activity restrictions   Pharmacologic therapy
                                   Follow-up care

PARASITIC DISORDERS

See also Developmental Problems/Needs.

Nursing Diagnoses

   Potential Alteration in Nutrition: Less Than Body
      Requirements, related to anorexia, nausea,
      vomiting, and deprivation of host nutrients by
      parasites
   Impairment of Skin Integrity related to pruritus
      secondary to emergence of parasites (pinworms)
      onto perianal skin, lytic necrosis, and tissue
      digestion
   Alteration in Bowel Elimination: Diarrhea, related to
      parasitic irritation to intestinal mucosa
   Alteration in Comfort: Abdominal Pain, related to
      parasitic invasion of small intestines
   Potential for Infection Transmission related to
      contagious nature of parasites
   Knowledge Deficit: (specify)
      Examples
         Condition
         Mode of transmission
         Prevention of reinfection
            Hygiene
            Clothing

POISONING

See also Dialysis, if indicated.
See also Unconscious Individual.

Collaborative Problems

Potential Complications
  Respiratory alkalosis   *Burns (acid/alkaline)*
  Metabolic acidosis   *Aspiration*
  Hemorrhage   *Blindness*
  Fluid/electrolyte
    imbalance

Nursing Diagnoses

Altered Comfort: Hyperpyrexia, related to heat production
    secondary to poisoning (*e.g.* salicylate)
Potential for Injury related to
  Examples
    Tonic/clonic movement   Bleeding tendencies
Anxiety/Fear related to invasive nature of treatments
    (gastric lavage, dialysis)
Anxiety (Parental) related to uncertainty of situation and
    feelings of guilt
Potential for Injury related to lack of awareness of
    environmental hazards
Knowledge Deficit: (specify)
  Examples
    Condition
    Treatments
    Home treatment of accidental poisoning
    Poison prevention
      Storage
      Teaching
      Poisonous plants
      Locks

RESPIRATORY TRACT INFECTION (Lower)

See also Developmental Problems/Needs.
See also Adult Pneumonia.

Collaborative Problems

Potential Complications
  Hyperthermia   *Septic shock*
  Respiratory insufficiency   *Paralytic ileus*

Nursing Diagnoses

Altered Comfort related to hyperthermia, malaise, and
    respiratory distress

Potential Alteration in Nutrition: Less Than Body
    Requirements, related to anorexia secondary to
    dyspnea and malaise

Anxiety related to breathlessness and apprehension

Potential Fluid Volume Deficit related to insufficient
    intake secondary to dyspnea and malaise

Potential Alteration in Body Temperature related to
    infectious process

Knowledge Deficit: (specify)
  Examples
    Condition
    Prevention of recurrence
    Treatment
      Oxygen
      Croup tent

RHEUMATIC FEVER

See also Developmental Problems/Needs.

Collaborative Problems

Potential Complications
  Endocarditis

Nursing Diagnoses

Diversional Activity Deficit related to prescribed bed rest

Alteration in Nutrition: Less Than Body Requirements,
    related to anorexia

Alteration in Comfort related to arthralgia

Potential for Injury related to choreic movements

Potential Noncompliance: Long-term Antibiotic Therapy,
    related to difficulty of maintaining preventive drug
    therapy when illness is resolved

Knowledge Deficit: (specify)
  Examples
    Condition
    Signs and symptoms of complications
    Long-term antibiotic therapy
    Prevention of recurence
    Risk factors (surgery; *e.g.,* dental)

RHEUMATOID ARTHRITIS (Juvenile)

See also Developmental Problems/Needs.
See also Corticosteroid Therapy.

Collaborative Problems

Potential Complications
   Pericarditis   *Iridocyclitis*

Nursing Diagnoses

Activity Intolerance related to fatigue and pain
Impaired Physical Mobility related to pain and restricted
    joint movement
Altered Comfort: Acute Pain, related to swollen, inflamed
    joints and restricted movement
Knowledge Deficit: (specify)
    Examples
        Condition   Rest versus activity
        Pharmacologic therapy   Myths
        Exercise program   Community resources

REYE SYNDROME

See also Unconscious Individual, if indicated.

Collaborative Problems

Potential Complications
   Renal failure   Shock
   Increased intracranial   Seizures
      pressure   Coma
   Fluid/electrolyte   Respiratory distress
      imbalance   Diabetes insipidus
   Hepatic failure

Nursing Diagnoses

Anxiety (parental) related to diagnosis and uncertain
    prognosis
Potential for Injury related to uncontrolled tonic/clonic
    movements
Potential for Infection related to invasive monitoring
    procedures
Altered Comfort related to hyperpyrexia and malaise
    secondary to disease process
Anxiety/Fear related to separation from family, sensory
    bombardment (ICU, treatments), and unfamiliar
    experiences

Alteration in Family Process related to
  Examples
    Critical nature of syndrome
    Hospitalization of child
    Separation of family members
Grieving related to actual, anticipated, or possible death
  of child
Potential Impairment of Skin Integrity related to
  immobility
Knowledge Deficit: (specify)
  Examples
    Condition
      Etiology
      Course
    Treatments
    Complications

SCOLIOSIS

See also Developmental Problems/Needs.

Nursing Diagnoses

Impaired Physical Mobility related to restricted
  movement secondary to braces
Potential Impairment of Skin Integrity related to
  mechanical irritation of brace
Potential Noncompliance related to chronicity and
  complexity of treatment regimen
Potential for Injury: Falls, related to restricted range of
  motion
Knowledge Deficit: (specify)
  Examples
    Condition
    Treatment
      Medical
      Surgical
    Exercises
    Environmental hazards
    Care of appliances
    Follow-up care
    Community services

SICKLE CELL ANEMIA

*See also Developmental Problems/Needs if the individual
is a child.*

Collaborative Problems

Potential Complications
Sickling crisis
Transfusion therapy

Thrombosis and infarction
Cholelithiasis

Nursing Diagnoses

Alteration in Tissue Perfusion: Peripheral, related to viscous blood and occulsion of microcirculation

Alteration in Comfort: Pain, related to viscous blood and tissue hypoxia

Self-care Deficit: (specify), related to pain and immobility of exacerbations

Knowledge Deficit: (specify)
Examples
Hazards
Signs and symptoms of complications

Fluid requirements
Hereditary factors

TONSILLITIS

See also Tonsillectomy, if indicated.

Collaborative Problems

Potential Complications
Otitis media
Rheumatic fever (β-hemolytic streptococci)

Nursing Diagnoses

Alteration in Comfort: Pain related to inflammation

Potential Fluid Volume Deficit related to inadequate fluid intake

Knowledge Deficit: (specify)
Examples
Condition
Treatments
Medical
Surgical
Nutritional/fluid requirements
Signs and symptoms of complications

WILMS' TUMOR

See also Developmental Problems/Needs.
See also Nephrectomy.
See also Cancer (General).

Collaborative Problems

Potential Complications
  Metastases to liver, lung, bone, brain
  Sepsis

Nursing Diagnoses

Potential for Injury related to rupture of tumor capsule
    secondary to manipulation/palpation of abdomen
Anxiety/Fear (child) related to
  Examples
    Age-related concerns
      Separation
      Strangers
      Pain
    Response of others to visible signs (alopecia)
    Uncertain future
Anxiety/Fear (parental) related to
  Examples
    Unknown prognosis   Treatments
    Painful procedures   (chemotherapy)
                               Feelings of inadequacy
Grieving related to actual, anticipated, or possible death
    of child
Spiritual Distress related to nature of disease and its
    possible disturbances on belief systems
Knowledge Deficit: (specify)
  Examples
    Condition   Nutritional
    Prognosis   requirements
    Treatments (side-effects) Follow-up care
    Home care   Community services

Psychiatric Disorders

AFFECTIVE DISORDERS (Depression)

Nursing Diagnoses

  Self-care Deficit: Grooming, related to decreased
    interest in body, inability to make decisions, and
    feelings of worthlessness

Ineffective Individual Coping: Anger, related to internal
conflicts (guilt, low self-esteem) or feelings of
rejection

Impaired Social Interactions related to alienation from
others by constant complaining, ruminations, or
loss of pleasure from relationships

Ineffective Individual Coping: Excessive Physical
Complaints (Without Organic Etiology), related to
inability to express emotional needs directly

Social Isolation related to inability to initiate activities
to reduce isolation secondary to low energy levels

Grieving: Pathological Pattern, related to unresolved
grief, prolonged denial, and repression

Disturbance in Self-concept related to feelings of
worthlessness and failure

Ineffective Family Coping related to marital discord
and role conflicts secondary to effects of chronic
depression

Powerlessness related to unrealistic negative beliefs
about self-worth or abilities

Alterations in Thought Processes related to negative
cognitive set (overgeneralizing, polarized thinking,
selected abstraction, arbitrary inference)

Sexual Dysfunction related to decreased sex drive, loss
of interest and pleasure

Diversional Activity Deficit related to a loss of interest
or pleasure in usual activities and low energy levels

Impaired Home Maintenance Management related to
inability to make decisions or concentrate

Potential for Self-harm related to feelings of
hopelessness and loneliness

Sleep Pattern Disturbance related to difficulty in falling
asleep or early morning awakening secondary to
emotional stress

Alteration in Bowel Elimination: Constipation, related
to sedentary life-style, insufficient exercise, or
inadequate diet

Potential Alteration in Nutrition: More Than Body
Requirements, related to increased intake versus
decreased activity expenditures secondary to
boredom and frustrations

Potential Alteration in Nutrition: Less Than Body

Requirements, related to anorexia secondary to
emotional stress
Knowledge Deficit: (specify)
Examples
Condition
Behavior modification
Therapy options
Pharmacologic
Electroshock
Community resources

ANOREXIA NERVOSA

Collaborative Problems

Potential Complications

Anemia   Cardiac dysrhythmias
Hypotension

Nursing Diagnoses

Alteration in Nutrition: Less Than Body Requirements,
related to anorexia and self-induced vomiting
following eating and laxative abuse
Disturbance in Self-concept related to inaccurate
perception of self as obese
Potential Fluid Volume Defici⁺ related to vomiting and
excessive weight loss
Sleep Pattern Disturbance related to fears and anxiety
concerning weight status
Activity Intolerance related to fatigue secondary to
malnutrition
Ineffective Individual Coping related to self-induced
vomiting, denial of hunger, and insufficient food
intake secondary to feelings of loss of control and
inaccurate preceptions of body states
Ineffective Family Coping related to marital discord and
its effect on family members
Potential Impairment of Skin Integrity related to dry skin
secondary to malnourished state
Alteration in Bowel Elimination: Constipation, related to
insufficient food and fluid intake
Impaired Social Interactions related to inability to form
relationships with others or fear of trusting
relationships with others

Fear of Sexuality, Maturity related to dissatisfaction with relationships with others (parents, peers)

ANXIETY AND ADJUSTMENT DISORDERS
(Phobias, Anxiety States, Traumatic Stress Disorders, Adjustment Reactions)

See also Substance Use Disorders, if indicated.

Nursing Diagnoses

Ineffective Individual Coping related to irrational avoidance of objects or situations

Impaired Social Interactions related to effects of behavior and actions on forming and maintaining relationships

Ineffective Individual Coping related to dependency on drugs

Anxiety related to irrational thoughts or guilt

Social Isolation related to irrational fear of social situations

Ineffective Individual Coping related to avoidance of objects or situations secondary to a numbing of responsiveness following a traumatic event

Sleep Pattern Disturbance related to recurrent nightmares

Disturbance in Self-concept related to feelings of guilt

Ineffective Individual Coping related to altered ability to constructively manage stressors secondary to (specify)

Examples

Physical illness	Natural disasters
Marital discord	Developmental crisis
Business crisis	

Knowledge Deficit

Examples

Condition

Pharmacologic therapy

Legal system regarding violence

BIPOLAR DISORDER (Mania)

Nursing Diagnoses

Disturbance in Self-concept related to exaggerated sense of self-importance and abilities secondary to feelings of inadequacy and inferiority

impaired Social Interaction related to overt hostility,
overconfidence, or manipulation of others
Potential for Violence to Others related to impaired
reality testing, impaired judgment, or inability to
control behavior
Sleep Pattern Disturbance related to hyperactivity
Alterations in Thought Process related to flight of ideas,
delusions, or hallucinations
Impaired Verbal Communication related to pressured
speech
Potential Fluid Volume Deficit related to altered
sodium excretion secondary to lithium therapy
Noncompliance related to feelings of no longer
requiring medication
Knowledge Deficit: (specify)
   Examples
      Condition
      Pharmacologic therapy

CHILDHOOD BEHAVIORAL DISORDERS
(Attention Deficit Disorders, Learning Disabilities)

Nursing Diagnoses

Alteration in Thought Process related to inattention
and impulsivity
Impaired Social Interactions related to inattention,
impulsivity, or hyperactivity
Ineffective Individual Coping related to
   Examples
      Temper outbursts   Mood lability
      Negativism   Stubborness
Grieving (parental) related to anticipated losses
secondary to condition
Alteration in Family Process related to adjustment
requirements for situation
   Examples
      Time   Physical care
      Energy   Prognosis
      Money
Potential for Violence related to impaired ability to
control aggression
Potential Impaired Home Maintenance Management
related to inadequate resources, inadequate,
housing or impaired caregivers

Potential Social Isolation (Child, Family) related to
disability and requirements for caregivers

Potential Alteration in Parenting: Abuse, Rejection, or
Overprotection, related to inadequate resources or
inadequate coping mechanisms

Disturbance in Self-concept related to effects of
limitations on achievement of developmental tasks

PARANOID DISORDERS

Nursing Diagnoses

Impaired Social Interactions related to feelings of
mistrust and suspicions of others

Ineffective Individual Coping: Denial, Projection,
related to inability to accept own feelings and
responsibility for actions secondary to low self-
esteem

Potential Alteration in Nutrition: Less Than Body
Requirements, related to reluctance to eat
secondary to fear of poisoning

Alteration in Thought Processes related to inability to
evaluate reality secondary to feelings of mistrust

Social Isolation related to fear and mistrust of situations
and others

PERSONALITY DISORDERS

Examples

Schizoid	Histrionic
Antisocial	Passive–aggressive
Borderline	Paranoid
Narcissistic	Schizotypal
Avoidant	Dependent
Compulsive	

Nursing Diagnoses

Ineffective Individual Coping: Passive Dependence
related to subordinating one's needs to decisions of
others

Ineffective Individual Coping:

Inappropriate intense anger

Lack of impulse control

Marked mood shifts

Habitual disregard for social norms related to altered
ability to meet responsibilities (role, social)

Impaired Social Interaction related to inability to
maintain enduring attachments secondary to
negative responses

Ineffective Individual Coping related to resistance
(procrastination, stubbornness, intentional
inefficiency) in responses to responsibilities (role,
social)

SCHIZOPHRENIC DISORDERS

Nursing Diagnoses

Alteration in Thought Processes related to inability to
evaluate reality

Potential for Violence to Others or Self-harm related to
responding to delusional thoughts or hallucinations

Impaired Verbal Communication related to incoherent/
illogical speech pattern, poverty of content of
speech, and side-effects of medications

Impaired Social Interactions related to

Examples

Withdrawal from	Inappropriate affect
External world	Inappropriate
Preoccupation	movements
with egocentric	Extreme
and illogical	suspiciousness
ideas	

Anxiety related to inability to cope with internal/
external stressors

Impaired Home Maintenance Management related to
impaired judgment, inability to self-initiate
activity, and loss of skills over long course of
illness

SOMATOFORM DISORDERS (Somatization,
Hypochondriasis, Conversion Reactions)

See also Affective Disorders, if indicated.

Nursing Diagnoses

Impaired Social Interactions related to the effects of
multiple somatic complaints on relationships

Ineffective Individual Coping related to unrealistic fear
of having a disease despite reassurance to contrary

Ineffective Individual Coping: Depression, related to belief of not getting proper care or sufficient response from others for complaints

Ineffective Family Coping related to chronicity of illness

Noncompliance related to impaired judgments and thought disturbances

Self-care Deficit: Dressing/Grooming, related to loss of skills and lack of interest in body and appearance

Social Isolation related to withdrawal from environment

Diversional Activity Deficit related to apathy, inability to initiate goal-directed activities, and loss of skills

Disturbance in Self-concept related to feelings of worthlessness and lack of ego boundaries

Knowledge Deficit: (specify)

Examples

Condition	Tardive dyskinesia
Pharmacologic therapy	Occupational skills
	Social skills

SUBSTANCE ABUSE DISORDERS

Nursing Diagnoses

Alteration in Nutrition: Less Than Body Requirements, related to anorexia

Potential Fluid Volume Deficit related to abnormal fluid loss secondary to vomiting and diarrhea

Potential for Injury related to disorientation, tremors, or impaired judgement

Potential for Self-harm related to disorientation, tremors, or impaired judgment

Potential for Violence related to

Examples

Impulsive behavior	Tremors
Disorientation	Impaired judgment

Sleep Pattern Disturbances related to irritability, tremors, and nightmares

Anxiety related to loss of control

Ineffective Individual Coping: Anger, Dependence, or Denial, related to inability to constructively manage stressors without drugs/alcohol

Sensory–Perceptual Alterations related to:

Examples
  Confusion   Impaired judgments
  Memory losses   Overdose/withdrawal
Disturbance in Self-concept related to guilt, mistrust, or
    ambivalence
Impaired Social Interactions related to
  Examples
    Emotional   High anxiety
      immaturity   Impulsive behavior
    Irritability   Aggressive responses
Social Isolation related to loss of work or withdrawal
    from others
Sexual Dysfunction related to impotence/loss of libido
    secondary to altered self-concept and substance
    abuse
Alteration in Family Processes related to disruption in
    marital dyad and inconsistent limit setting
Knowledge Deficit: (specify)
  Examples
    Condition   High-risk situations
    Treatments available   Community
                                 resources

Diagnostic and Therapeutic Procedures

ANGIOPLASTY (Percutaneous, Transluminal,
Coronary, Peripheral)

Preprocedure Period
Nursing Diagnoses
Knowledge Deficit: (specify)
  Examples
    Procedure
    Preparation
    Postprocedure care
Anxiety/Fear related to procedure, outcome, and
    possible need for surgery

Postprocedure Period

Collaborative Problems

Potential Complications
  Dysrhythmias (coronary)
  Acute coronary occlusion (clot, spasm, collapse)
  Myocardial infarction (coronary)
  Arterial dissection or rupture
  Hemorrhage/hematoma (site)
  Paresthesia distal to site
  Arterial thrombosis
  Embolization (peripheral)

Nursing Diagnoses

Impaired Physical Mobility related to prescribed
    immobility and restricted movement of involved
    extremity
Knowledge Deficit: (specify)
  Examples
    Condition   Medications
    Home activities   Signs and symptoms of
    Diet   complications

ANTICOAGULANT THERAPY

Collaborative Problems

Potential Complications
  Hemorrhage

Nursing Diagnoses

Knowledge Deficit: (specify)
  Examples
    Administration schedule
    Identification medallion/card
    Contraindications
      Foods   Medications
    Signs and symptoms of bleeding
      Skin   Gastrointestinal
      Neurological
    Potential hazards
      Surgery   Pregnancy
      Dental extraction   Shaving

ARTERIOGRAM

Preprocedure Period
Nursing Diagnoses
Knowledge Deficit: (specify)
  Examples
    Procedure
      Equipment
      Possible sensations
    Preparation
    Post-care

Postprocedure Period
Collaborative Problems
Potential Complications

Hematoma formation	Paresthesia
Hemorrhage	Embolism
Stroke	Allergic reaction

CARDIAC CATHETERIZATION

Preprocedure Period
Nursing Diagnoses
Knowledge Deficit: (specify)
  Examples
    Procedure
      Purpose
      Appearance of laboratory, positioning
      Equipment
      Length
      Possible sensations
    Preparation
      NPO
      Premedication
    Postprocedure care (frequent vs. activity
      restriction)
  Anxiety/Fear related to being awake during the
    procedure

Postprocedure Period
Collaborative Problems
Potential Complications
  Systemic (hypovolemia/hypervolemia, allergic reaction)

Cardiac (arrhythmias, myocardial infarction, perforation)
Cerebrovascular accident (CVA)
Neurovascular (hematoma formation [site], hemorrhage
[site], paresis, or paresthesia)

Nursing Diagnoses

Alteration in Comfort related to tissue trauma and
prescribed postprocedure immobilization

CASTS

Collaborative Problems

Potential Complications
Pressure (edema, mechanical)
Compartmental syndrome
Ulcer formation
Infection

Nursing Diagnoses

Potential for Injury related to hazards of crutch walking
and impaired mobility secondary to cast

Potential Impairment of Skin Integrity related to pressure
of cast on skin surface

Potential Impaired Home Maintenance Management
related to the restrictions imposed by cast on
performing activities of daily living and role
responsibilities

Self-care Deficits: (specify), related to limitation of
movement secondary to cast

Potential Alteration in Respiratory Function related to
imposed immobility or restricted respiratory
movement secondary to cast (body)

Diversional Activity Deficit related to boredom and
inability to perform usual recreational activities

Knowledge Deficit: (specify)
Examples
Crutch-walking
Cast care
Exercise program
Signs and symptoms of complications

Numbness	Cyanosis
Tingling	Odor or pain

| Burning | Inability to move |
| Blanching | distal parts |

CHEMOTHERAPY

See also Cancer (General).

Collaborative Problems

Potential Complications

Necrosis/phlebitis at	Peripheral nerve toxicosis
intravenous site	Anaphylaxis
Thrombocytopenia	Pulmonary fibrosis
Anemia	Central nervous system
Leukopenia	toxicity

Nursing Diagnoses

Potential Fluid Volume Deficit related to gastrointestinal fluid losses secondary to vomiting

Alteration in Nutrition: Less Than Body Requirements, related to anorexia, nausea, and altered taste sensations

Potential for Infection related to altered immune system secondary to effects of cytotoxic agents or disease process

Activity Intolerance related to fatigue

Potential Alteration in Family Processes related to interruptions imposed by treatment and schedule on patterns of living

Potential Sexual Dysfunction related to amenorrhea and sterility (temporary/permanent) secondary to effects of chemotherapy on testes/ovaries

Potential for Injury related to bleeding tendencies

Alteration in Bowel Elimination: Constipation/Diarrhea, related to decreased bowel activity or irritation of epithelium of bowel

Alteration in Oral Mucous Membrane related to irritation of mucosa from medication

CORTICOSTEROID THERAPY

Collaborative Problems

Potential Complications

| Peptic ulcer | Hypertension |

Diabetes mellitus   *Thromboembolism*
Osteoporosis   *Hypokalemia*

Nursing Diagnoses

Potential Fluid Volume Excess: Edema, related to sodium
    and water retention
Potential for Infection related to immunosuppression
    secondary to excessive adrenocortical hormones
Potential Alteration in Nutrition: More Than Body
    Requirements, related to increased appetite
Disturbance in Self-concept related to appearance changes
    (*e.g.,* abnormal fat distribution, increased production
    of androgens)
Knowledge Deficit: (specify)
  Examples
    Administration schedule
    Indications for therapy
    Side-effects
    Signs and symptoms of complications
    Hazards of adrenal insufficiency
    Potential causes of adrenal insufficiency
      Injuries   Abrupt cessation of
      Surgery   therapy
      Vomiting
    Emergency kit
    Dietary requirements
    Prevention of infection

GASTROSTOMY

Collaborative Problems

Potential Complications
  Gastrointestinal bleeding

Nursing Diagnoses

Potential for Infection related to gastrostomy incision and
    enzymatic action of gastric juices on skin
Altered Comfort: Pain, related to incision and tension on
    gastrostomy tube
Potential Alteration in Nutrition: Less Than Body
    Requirements, related to intake dependent on
    gastrostomy feedings
Potential Disturbance in Self-concept related to inability
    to taste or swallow food/liquids

Knowledge Deficit: (specify)
  Examples
    Nutritional requirements
    Home care
    Signs and symptoms of complications
        Infection
        Weight loss
        Nonpatent gastrostomy tube
        Diarrhea

HEMODIALYSIS

See also Chronic Renal Failure.

Collaborative Problems

Potential Complications (During/After Treatment)

Fluid imbalances (disequilibrium syndrome)
Electrolyte imbalance (potassium, sodium)
Nausea/vomiting
Transfusion reaction
Aneurysm
Hemorrhage
Vascular access (fistulas, graft, shunts, venous catheters)
Bleeding
Dialysate leakage
Clots
Disconnection
Infection
Hepatitis B
Fever/chills

Nursing Diagnoses

Potential for Injury to (Vascular) Access Site related to vulnerability
Potential for Infection related to direct access to bloodstream secondary to vascular access
Powerlessness related to need for treatments to live despite effects on life-style
Alteration in Family Processes related to the interruptions of treatment schedule on role responsibilities
Knowledge Deficit: (specify)
  Examples
    Rationale of treatment
    Access site
        Care (general, posttreatment)
        Precautions
        Emergency treatments (disconnected, bleeding, clotting)

Pretreatment instructions
   Dietary   Medications
Assessments
   Bruit   Weights
   Blood pressure

HEMODYNAMIC MONITORING

See also Medical Diagnosis of the individual.

Collaborative Problems

Potential Complications
  Sepsis
  Hemorrhage (site)
  Emboli
  Thrombosis (clotting)
  Bleeding back
  Vasospasm
  Tissue ischemia/hypoxia
  System problems (leaks, air bubbles, misconnection,
     damaged/unbalanced transducer, damaged
     amplifier, damaged stopcock, flush device, or
     pressure tubing)

Nursing Diagnoses

Potential for Infection related to direct access to
  bloodstream
Impaired Physical Mobility related to position restrictions
  during monitoring
Knowledge Deficit: (specify)
  Examples
    Purpose
    Procedure
    Associated care

HICKMAN CATHETER

Collaborative Problems

Potential Complications
  Air embolism   *Nonpatent catheter*

Nursing Diagnoses

Potential for Infection related to direct access to
  bloodstream

Potential Impaired Home Maintenance Management
related to lack of knowledge of catheter management

INTRA-AORTIC BALLOON PUMPING

Preprocedure Period
Nursing Diagnoses

Knowledge Deficit: (specify)
Examples
Procedure (preparation)
Nursing care

Intraprocedure/Postprocedure Period
Collaborative Problems

Potential Complications
Death
Arterial insufficiency/
thrombosis
Sepsis/infection
Peripheral neuropathy/
claudication
Thrombocytopenia
Bleeding
Emboli
Gastrointestinal bleeding
Disseminated
intravascular
coagulation
Mechanical malfunction
Dysrhythmias

Nursing Diagnoses

Impaired Physical Mobility related to prescribed
immobility and restricted movement of involved
extremity
Potential for Infection related to direct access to
bloodstream
Potential Alteration in Bowel Elimination: Constipation,
related to immobility and restricted movement of
involved limb
Potential Sensory–Perceptual Alterations related to:
Examples
Immobility
Pain
Excessive
environmental
stimuli
Disruption of
biorhythms
Anxiety/Fear related to treatments, environment, and risk
of death

Alteration in Family Processes related to the critical
nature of situation and uncertain prognosis

MECHANICAL VENTILATION

Collaborative Problems

Potential Complications
Acidosis/alkalosis
Disconnected ventilator
Airway obstruction/
atelectasis
Tracheal necrosis

Infection
Gastrointestinal bleeding
Tension pneumothorax
Oxygen toxicity
Respirator dependency

Nursing Diagnoses

Impaired Verbal Communication related to inability to
speak secondary to intubation

Potential Impairment of Skin Integrity related to imposed
immobility

Potential for Infection related to disruption of skin layer
secondary to tracheostomy

Alterations in Family Processes related to critical nature
of situation and uncertain prognosis

Anxiety/Fear related to condition, treatments,
environment, and risk of death

Potential Sensory–Perceptual Alterations related to
excessive environmental stimuli and decreased input
of meaningful stimuli secondary to treatment and
critical care unit

Powerlessness related to respirator dependency

PACEMAKER INSERTION

Preprocedure Period
Nursing Diagnoses

Knowledge Deficit: (specify)
Examples
Procedure
Purpose
Appearance of operating room/laboratory
Positioning
Equipment
Possible sensations

Preparation
  Skin preparation
  Premedication
  NPO status
Postprocedure
  X-rays
  Electrocardiograms
  Vital signs
  Monitoring
  Activity restrictions
  Site care

Postprocedure Period
Collaborative Problems

Potential Complications
  Cardiac (perforation, dysrhythmias)
  *Pacemaker (failure, electromagnetic interference, under/
    oversensing, partial/improper sensing or wire break)*
  Rejection of unit
  Pressure necrosis of skin over unit
  Site (hemorrhage, infection)

Nursing Diagnoses

Altered Comfort related to pain at insertion site and
  prescribed postprocedure immobilization
Potential Alteration in Respiratory Function related to
  imposed postprocedure immobility
Potential for Infection related to operative site
Knowledge Deficit. (specify)
  Examples
    Site care
    Signs and symptoms of skin complications
    Electromagnetic interference

Microwave ovens	Electric motors
Arc welding	Antitheft devices
equipment	Power transmitters
Gasoline engines	

    Pacemaker function
      Daily pulse taking
      Signs of impending battery failure
    Activity restrictions
    Follow-up care

PERITONEAL DIALYSIS

Collaborative Problems

Potential Complications
  Fluid imbalances
  Electrolyte imbalances
  Hemorrhage
  Negative nitrogen balance
  Catheter problems (displacement, plugging, fibrin clots)
  Bowel/bladder perforation
  Hyperglycemia
  Peritonitis

Nursing Diagnoses

Potential for Infection related to direct access to
    peritoneal cavity, need to disconnect catheter for
    treatment, and growth medium potential of the
    dialysate (high glucose concentration)
Potential for Injury to catheter site related to vulnerability
Potential Impaired Breathing Patterns related to
    immobility and pressure on diaphragm during dwell
    time
Altered Comfort related to
  Examples
    Rapid instillation
    Pressure from fluid
    Excessive suction during outflow
    Extreme temperature of solution (hot or cold)
Potential Alteration in Nutrition: Less Than Body
    Requirements, related to anorexia secondary to
    abdominal distention during dialysis, protein loss in
    dialysate, or vomiting
Potential Fluid Volume Excess related to fluid retention
    secondary to catheter problems (kinks, blockages)
    and/or position
Alteration in Family Processes related to interruptions of
    treatment schedule on role responsibilities
Powerlessness related to need for treatment to live despite
    effects on life-style
Impaired Home Maintenance Management related to lack
    of knowledge of treatment procedure
Knowledge Deficit: (specify)

Examples
    Rationale of treatment
    Home care
    Self-care activities
        Protection of catheter
        Aseptic technique
    Activity needs
    Prescribed diet
    Control of fluid intake/output
    Medication regimen
    Signs/symptoms of complications
    Follow-up visits
    Daily recording
        Intake
        Output
        Blood pressure
        Weights

RADIATION THERAPY (External)

Pre–therapy Period
Nursing Diagnoses

Knowledge Deficit: (specify)
    Examples
        Procedure
        Site-related, local/systemic effects of therapy (skin
            gastrointestinal, neurologic, oral membranes)

Post–therapy Period
Collaborative Problem

Potential Complication of Head/Brain Irradiation
    Increased intracranial pressure

Nursing Diagnoses

Potential Impairment of Skin Integrity related to radiation
    exposure
Disturbance in Self-concept related to alopecia secondary
    to irradiation to head and visible markings outlining
    treatment field
Alteration in Oral Mucous Membrane related to
    mucositis, gingivitis, esophagitis, and dry mouth
    secondary to irradiation (head/neck, chest/back)

Altered Comfort related to nausea and vomiting
secondary to irradiation of abdomen/lower back
Alteration in Bowel Elimination: Diarrhea, related to
increased peristalsis secondary to irradiation of
abdomen/lower back
Potential for Infection: Skin, related to moist skin reaction
Potential Alteration in Nutrition: Less Than Body
Requirements, related to anorexia, nausea/vomiting,
or stomatitis
Activity Intolerance related to fatigue secondary to
treatments or transportation
Knowledge Deficit: (specify)
Examples
Skin care
Signs of complications

TOTAL PARENTERAL NUTRITION
(Hyperalimentation Therapy)

Collaborative Problems

Potential Complications
Sepsis
Hypoglycemia/
hyperglycemia
Air embolism

Perforation
Pneumothorax,
hydrothorax,
hemothorax

Nursing Diagnoses

Potential for Infection related to catheter's direct access to
bloodstream
Potential Impairment of Skin Integrity related to
continuous skin surface irritation secondary to
catheter and adhesive
Potential Disturbance in Self-concept related to inability
to ingest food
Potential Alteration in Oral Mucous Membrane related to
inability to ingest food/fluid
Knowledge Deficit: (specify)
Examples
Home care
Signs and symptoms of complications
Catheter care
Follow-up care (laboratory studies)

Appendix

Adult Data-Base Assessment Guide

This guide directs the nurse to collect data to assess functional health patterns* of the individual and to determine the presence of actual, potential, or possible nursing diagnoses. When the person has a medical problem, the nurse will also have to assess for data in order to collaborate with the physician in monitoring the problem.

As with any printed assessment tool, the nurse must determine whether to collect or defer collecting certain data. The symbol △ identifies data that should be collected on hospitalized persons. The collection of data in sections not marked with △ should probably be deferred with most acutely ill persons or when the information is irrelevant to the individual.

As the nurse interviews the person, significant data may surface. The nurse should then ask other questions (focus assessment) to determine the presence of a pattern. For further information, the reader is referred to Section II of *Nursing Diagnosis: Application to Clinical Practice*, 2nd ed., by Lynda Juall Carpenito (Philadelphia, JB Lippincott, 1987).

For example, the client reports during the initial interview that she has a problem with incontinence. The nurse should then ask specific questions utilizing the focus assessment for Alteration in Patterns of Urinary Elimination to deter-

* The functional health patterns have been adapted from Gordon M: Nursing Diagnosis: Application and Process. New York, McGraw-Hill, 1982.

mine which diagnosis of incontinence is present. After the nurse has identified the factors, the plan of care can be initiated.

Data-Base Assessment Format

1. Health perception–health management pattern
   A. Health management

   "How would you usually describe your health?"

Excellent	Fair
Good	Poor

   "How would you describe your health at this time?"

   Review the daily health practices of the individual (adults, children).

Dental care	Exercise regimen
Food intake	Leisure activities
Fluid intake	Responsibility in the family

   Use of

Tobacco	Alcohol
Salt, sugar, fat products	Drugs (over-the-counter, prescribed)

   Knowledge of safety practices

Fire prevention	Automobile (maintenance, seatbelts)
Water safety	
Children	
	Bicycle
	Poison control

   Knowledge of disease and preventive behavior

   Specific diseases (*e.g.,* heart disease, cancer, respiratory disease, childhood diseases, infections, dental disease)

   Susceptibility (*e.g.,* presence of risk factors, family history)

   "What do you do to keep healthy and to prevent disorders in yourself? In your children?"

Adequate nutrition	Professional examinations (gynecological, dental)
Weight control	
Exercise program	
Self-examinations (breasts, testicles)	Immunizations

B. Developmental History*

Family history (diagrammatic outline of family
structure, indicating illnesses of living;
deceased; cause and age)

Maternal   Parental grandparents
grandparents   Father
Mother   Siblings
Spouse

Patient
Children

Assess for achievement of developmental tasks.

Young adult

(Intimacy vs. isolation)

Accepting self and stabilizing self-concept

Establishing independence from parental home
and financial aid

Becoming established in a vocation or profession
that provides personal satisfaction,
economic independence, and a feeling of
making a worthwhile contribution to
society

Learning to appraise and express love,
responsibility through more than sexual
contexts

Establishing an intimate bond with another,
either through marriage or with a close
friend

Establishing and managing a residence, home

Finding a congenial social group

Deciding whether to have children

Formulating a meaningful philosophy of life

Becoming involved as a citizen in the
community

Middle age

(Generativity vs. stagnation)

Developing a sense of unity and abiding
intimacy with mate

Helping growing and grown children become
happy and responsible adults—
relinquishing central position in their life

* From Nursing History Guide, Nursing Department, Southeast-
ern Missouri University, Cape Giraudeau, Missouri

Taking pride in accomplishments of self and spouse

Finding pleasure in generativity and recognition in work

Balancing work with other roles

Preparing for retirement

Role reversal with parents—parental loss

Achieving mature social and civic responsibility

Develop or maintain active organizational membership

Accept and adjust to changes of middle age (physical)

Socialization with new and old friends

Use of leisure time

Older adult

(Integrity vs. despair)

Decide how and where to live out remaining years

Continue supportive, close, and warm relationship with significant others including a satisfying sexual relationship, if desired

Satisfactory living arrangements—safe, comfortable household routine

Supplemental retirement income if possible

Maintain maximal level of self–health care

Maintain interest in people outside of family

Maintain social, civic, and political responsibility

Pursue interests

Finding meaning in life after retirement

Facing inevitable illness and death of self and significant others

Formulating a philosophy of life

Finding meaning to life through philosophy/ religion

Adjusting to death of spouse or other loved one

C. Health perception

△ Reason for and expectations of hospitalization (and previous hospital experiences)

△ "Describe your illness."

    Cause   Onset

△ "What treatments or practices have been prescribed?"

Diet	Surgery
Weight loss	Cessation of
Medications	smoking
	Exercises

△ "Have you been able to follow the prescribed instructions?" If not, "What has prevented you?"

△ "Have you experienced or do you anticipate a problem with caring for yourself (your children, your home)?"

Mobility	Financial
problems	concerns
Sensory	Structural
deficits	barriers
(vision,	(stairs,
hearing)	narrow
	doorways)

△ "Are there any problems that could contribute to falls or accidents?"

    Unfamiliar setting

    Decreased sensorium (vertigo, confusion)

    Sensory deficits (visual, auditory, tactile)

    Motor deficits (gait, tremors, range of motion, coordination)

    Urinary/bowel urgency

2. △ Nutritional–metabolic pattern

"What is the usual daily food intake (meals, snacks)?"

"What is the usual fluid intake (type, amounts)?"

"How is your appetite?"

Indigestion	Vomiting
Nausea	Sore mouth

"What are your food restrictions or preferences?"

"Any supplements (vitamins, feedings)?"

"Has your weight changed in the past 6 months?" If yes, "Why? How much?"

"Any problems with ability to eat?"

Swallow liquids	Chew
Swallow solids	Feed self

Skin

"What is the skin condition?"

Color, temperature, turgor	Edema (type, location)
Lesions (type, description, location)	Pruritus (location)

△ "Are there any factors present that could contribute to pressure ulcer development?"

Immobility	Dehydration
Malnourished	Decreased circulation
Sensory deficits	

3. △ Elimination pattern

Bladder

"Are there any problems or complaints with the usual pattern of urinating?"

Oliguria	Retention
Polyuria	Burning
Dysuria	Incontinence
Dribbling	

"Do you use assistive devices?"

Intermittent catheterization	Incontinence briefs
	Cystostomy
Catheter (Foley, external)	

Bowel

"What is the usual time, frequency, color, consistency, pattern?"

"Assistive devices (type, frequency)?"

Ileostomy	Cathartics
Colostomy	Laxatives
Enemas	Suppositories

4. Activity–exercise pattern

"Describe usual daily/weekly activities of daily living."

Occupation	Exercise pattern
Leisure activities	(type, frequency)

△ "Are there any limitations in ability?"

Ambulating (gait, weight-bearing, balance)
Bathing self (shower, tub)
Dressing/grooming (oral hygiene)
Toileting (commode, toilet, bedpan)

"Are there complaints of dyspnea or fatigue?"

△ "Are there factors present that could interfere with
    self-care after discharge?"

Motor deficits	Cognitive/sensory
Emotional deficits	deficits
Lack of knowledge	Environmental
	barriers
	Lack of resources

5. △ Sleep–rest pattern
   "What is the usual sleep pattern?"

Bedtime	Sleep aids
Hours slept	(medication,
	food)
	Sleep routine

   "Any problems?"

Difficulty falling	Not feeling rested
asleep	after sleep
Difficulty remaining	
asleep	

6. △ Cognitive–perceptual pattern
   "Any deficits in sensory perception (hearing, sight,
      touch)?"

Glasses	Hearing aid

   "Any complaints?"

Vertigo	Insensitivity to cold
Insensitivity to	or heat
superficial pain	

   "Able to read and write?"
7. Self-perception pattern
      △ "What are you most concerned about?"
      "What are your present health goals?"
      △ "How would you describe yourself?"
      "Has being ill made you feel different about
         yourself?"
      "To what do you attribute the following?"

Becoming ill	Maintaining health
Getting better	

8. Role-relationship pattern
   △ Communication
   "Any hearing deficits?" (aids, lip-reads)
   "What language do you speak?"
   "Is speech clear? Relevant?"
   Assess ability to express self and understand others
      (orally, in writing, with gestures)

Relationships

"Do you live alone?" If not, "With whom?"

"Whom do you turn to for help in time of need?"

Assess family life (members, educational level, occupations)

Cultural background	Decision-making
Activities (lone or group)	Communication patterns
Role discipline	Finances

"Any complaints?"

Parenting difficulties	Marital difficulties
Difficulties with relatives (in-laws, parents)	Abuse (physical, verbal, substance)

9. Sexuality–sexual functioning

"Has there been or do you anticipate a change in your sexual relations because of your condition?"

Fertility	Pregnancy
Libido	Contraceptives
Erections	
Menstruation	

Assess knowledge of sexual functioning

10. Coping–stress management pattern

△ "How do you make decisions (alone, with assistance, with whom)?"

△ "Has there been a loss in your life in the past year (or changes—moves, job, health)?"

"What do you like about yourself?"

"What would you like to change in your life?"

"What is preventing you?"

"What do you do when you are tense or under stress (e.g., problem-solve, eat, sleep, take medication, seek help)?"

△ "What can the nurses do to provide you with more comfort and security during your hospitalization?"

11. Value–belief system

"With what (whom) do you find a source of strength or meaning?"

"Is religion or God important to you?"

"What are your religious practices (type, frequency)?"

"Have your values or moral beliefs been challenged
    recently? Describe."
Δ "Is there a religious person or practice (diet, book,
    ritual) that you would desire during
    hospitalization (institutionalization)?"

12. Δ Physical assessment (objective)
  General appearance
  Weight and height
  Eyes (appearance, drainage)
    Pupils (size: equal; reactive to light)
    Vision (glasses)
  Mouth
    Mucous membrane (color, moisture, lesions)
    Teeth (condition: loose, broken; dentures)
  Hearing (hearing aids)
  Pulses (radial, apical, peripheral)
    Rate, rhythm, volume
  Respirations
    Rate, quality, breath sounds (upper and lower
      lobes)
  Blood pressure
  Temperature
  Skin (color, temperature, turgor)
    Lesions, edema, pruritus
  Functional ability (mobility and safety)
    Dominant hand
    Use of right and left hands, arms, legs
    Strength, grasp
    Range of motion
    Gait (stability)
    Use of aids (wheelchair, braces, cane, walker)
    Weight-bearing (full, partial, none)
  Mental status
    Orientation (time, place, person, events)
    Memory
    Affect
    Eye contact

Index

Nursing diagnostic categories appear in **boldface**.